Planning and Care for Children and Adolescents with Dental Enamel Defects

Bernadette K. Drummond
Nicola Kilpatrick

Editors

Planning and Care for Children and Adolescents with Dental Enamel Defects

Etiology, Research and Contemporary Management

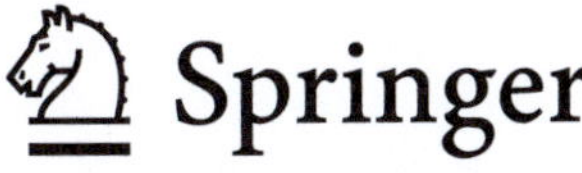 Springer

Editors
Bernadette K. Drummond, BDS, MS, PhD
Oral Sciences
University of Otago School of Dentistry
Dunedin
New Zealand

Nicola Kilpatrick, BDS, PhD
Cleft and Craniofacial Research
Murdoch Childrens Research Institute
Melbourne Victoria
Australia

ISBN 978-3-662-51313-2   ISBN 978-3-662-44800-7   (eBook)
DOI 10.1007/978-3-662-44800-7
Springer Heidelberg New York Dordrecht London

Preface

The prevalence of developmental defects of enamel (DDE) is reportedly increasing worldwide. It is difficult to assess this accurately, as in the past the greater prevalence of dental caries may have had a significant impact on the diagnosis of DDE by masking its presence. Clinically, defects vary greatly in their appearance in terms of size, color, and shape. DDE may affect both primary and permanent dentitions and can be either generalized across one or both dentitions or localized to specific teeth. The structure of enamel in affected teeth differs, such that there may be a quantitative reduction in enamel (known as hypoplasia) or a qualitative defect (known as hypomineralization), though often defects comprise a combination of the two. Despite the growing burden associated with treating affected individuals, there remains a lack of understanding of the etiology of DDE and evidence of clinical outcomes to support management.

When clinicians are faced with a child who has hypomineralized and/or hypoplastic teeth, it can be difficult to plan care for many reasons. Often, the child is young and has had little or no experience of dentistry. Apart from the difficulties for the child, this creates stress for the parents and puts pressure on clinicians trying to decide on the best way to manage the young patient. Affected teeth are difficult to anesthetize, and treatment can be uncomfortable. It is also clear that individuals with teeth affected by DDE experience significantly more restorative procedures throughout childhood and adolescence and have higher levels of dental anxiety. Poor esthetics coupled with increased sensitivity may further exacerbate the child's anxiety and have a real impact on their quality of life. Parents report that children eat slowly or refuse some foods, although they often do not complain directly of pain. Children note that they cannot eat ice cream or that people, including teachers and peers, comment on their chalky or discolored anterior teeth.

The protein content in hypomineralized enamel is significantly higher than in otherwise healthy enamel, which in turn alters its structure and interferes with the adhesion of conventional resin-based dental restorative materials. When a clinician looks at affected teeth for the first time, they should be aware that the child is likely to require a lifetime of care, even if the teeth remain caries free. This can be an overwhelming prospect when considering the best approach to early management so as to prepare the individual for the longer-term definitive solutions, which often cannot be finally decided until the child is in late adolescence or early adulthood. When severe defects are localized to one or only a few posterior teeth, it may be appropriate to extract these compromised teeth. However, it is important to consider the impact of such extractions on the developing occlusion in order to optimize definitive occlusal outcomes. Finally, there are financial considerations to be taken into account both immediately and in the long term, which also will impact on the management choices that families will be able to make.

With all this in mind, the aims of this book are to summarize the current understanding of DDE in the primary and permanent dentitions, to discuss its impact on children and adolescents, and to provide guidance on treatment planning and management. The prevalence and etiology of DDE are addressed in Chaps. 1, 2, and 3. Chapters 4 and 5 review the contemporary understanding of the genetic influences on DDE and the potential associations of DDE with systemic conditions and syndromes. Dental professionals can play an important role in the diagnosis of systemic conditions if they record patterns of defects and take careful histories of other related health signs and symptoms. Chapter 6 is devoted to presenting information on the structure and composition of defective enamel. This is to encourage clinicians to think about how affected teeth behave in the oral environment and consider the impact of this on restorative materials and treatment techniques. Affected teeth pose particular challenges in relation to resin bonding, and clinicians have to consider where to place restoration margins and whether/how to pretreat the enamel to improve adhesion.

Chapter 7 summarizes the current knowledge of the impact of DDE from the patient's perspective. There is emerging awareness of the impact of DDE on children's and adolescents' quality of life not only in terms of the psychosocial influences of altered appearance but also as a result of a young person's experience of complex and often repeated dental interventions. This chapter highlights the importance of giving careful consideration to planning not only the obvious clinical treatment needs but also the longer-term treatment needs in the context of the broader psychosocial demands and individual/family expectations.

In planning a definitive outcome, clinicians have to consider the implications of growth on the developing occlusion, particularly where teeth have a very poor prognosis and extractions are being considered. Chapter 8 reviews dental and occlusal development. While specialist orthodontic input is ideal, this chapter also acknowledges that this is not always possible and gives an overview of the aspects of occlusion that should be considered when making decisions surrounding the choice and timing of extractions. The first chapter looking at the management of DDE (Chap. 9) is devoted to managing sensitivity, improving enamel mineralization, and preventing dental caries and erosion in affected teeth. Two Chaps. (10 and 11) address the immediate and intermediate restorative management of primary and permanent teeth with DDE. This includes the management of permanent teeth through adolescence, while planning the permanent restoration options. All these chapters give options and recommendations that are supported, where available, with contemporary evidence. The final chapter (Chap. 12) offers an interesting glimpse into cutting-edge research, in which techniques to regenerate enamel and develop enamel–like restorative materials offer hope for the future. As access to research reporting becomes increasingly available to all clinicians, this chapter is a guide on what to continue to search for in the future.

This book is intended to provide contemporary information on both DDE and its impact during childhood. Each of the chapters covering specific aspects of DDE has been written to stand alone. However, where appropriate, the reader is directed to further linked information in other chapters. Although guidance is offered on various management options from both preventive and restorative perspectives, it is not intended to suggest that these are the only options. Clinicians are encouraged to use the information to consider the best pathway for each individual patient after taking account of the child's and family's perspectives, the developing occlusion, the clinician's own skills, and the severity of the presenting anomaly.

Dunedin, New Zealand
Melbourne, Australia
Bernadette Kathleen Drummond, BDS, MS, PhD
Nicky Kilpatrick, BDS, PhD

Acknowledgements

Professor J. Kirkham for her insights into Chap. 13.
Dr. Supriya Raj for her amazing work organizing the references throughout the book.

Contents

Contributors

Robert P. Anthonappa, BDS, MDS, PhD Department of Paediatric Dentistry, School of Dentistry, Faculty of Medicine, Dentistry and Health Sciences, University of Western Australia, Perth, WA, Australia

Lucy A.L. Burbridge, BDS, DipConSed, MClinDent Paediatric Dental Department, Newcastle Dental Hospital, Newcastle Upon Tyne, UK

Angus Cameron, BDS, MDSc Department of Pediatric Dentistry, Westmead Hospital and The University of Sydney, Westmead, NSW, Australia

Sywe-Ren Chang, MS Department of Cariology, Restorative Sciences and Endodontics, School of Dentistry, University of Michigan, Ann Arbor, MI, USA

Brian H. Clarkson, BChD, MS, PhD Department Of Cariology, Restorative Sciences and Endodontics, School of Dentistry, University of Michigan, Ann Arbor, MI, USA

Felicity Crombie, BDSc (Hons), PhD Growth and Development Unit, Melbourne Dental School, University of Melbourne, Melbourne, VIC, Australia

Agata Czajka-Jakubowska, PhD Department of Maxillofacial Orthopedics and Orthodontics, Poznan University of Medical Sciences, Poznan, Poland

Bernadette K. Drummond, BDS, MS, PhD Department of Oral Sciences, Faculty of Dentistry, University of Otago, Dunedin, New Zealand

Monty Duggal, BDS, MDSc, PhD Department of Paediatric Dentistry, School of Dentistry, University of Leeds, Leeds, West Yorkshire, UK

Marlies E.C. Elfrink, PhD Paediatric dentist Mondzorgcentrum Nijverdal and member Paediatric REsearch Project (PREP), Department of Cariology Endodontology Pedodontology, Academic Centre for Dentistry (ACTA), Amsterdam, The Netherlands

Rami Farah, BDS, MPhil, DClinDent, PhD Department of Oral Sciences, Faculty of Dentistry, University of Otago, Dunedin, New Zealand

Suzanne M. Hanlin, BDS, MDS, GradDipHealInf Department of Oral Rehabilitation, University of Otago, Dunedin, New Zealand

Winifred Harding, BDS, MDS Department of Oral Sciences,
Discipline of Orthodontics, Faculty of Dentistry,
University of Otago, Dunedin, New Zealand

Mike Harrison, BDS, MScD, MPhil Department of Pediatric Dentistry,
Guy's and St Thomas' Dental Institute, London, UK

Nicky Kilpatrick, BDS, PhD Cleft and Craniofacial Research,
Murdoch Childrens Research Institute, Melbourne, VIC, Australia

Nigel M. King, BDS Hons, MSc Hons, PhD Department of Paediatric Dentistry,
School of Dentistry, Faculty of Medicine, Dentistry and Health Sciences,
University of Western Australia, Perth, WA, Australia

Jun Liu, PhD Department of Cariology, Restorative Sciences and Endodontics,
School of Dentistry, University of Michigan, Ann Arbor, MI, USA

Erin K. Mahoney, BDS, MDSc PhD Department of Dentistry,
Hutt Valley District Health Board, Wellington, New Zealand

David John Manton, BDSc, MDSc, PhD Growth and Development Unit,
Melbourne Dental School, University of Melbourne, VIC, Australia

Zoe Marshman, BDS, MPH, DDPH, PhD Academic Unit of Dental Public
Health, School of Clinical Dentistry, University of Sheffield, Claremont Crescent,
Sheffield, South Yorkshire, UK

Hani Nazzal, BDS, PhD Department of Paediatric Dentistry, School of Dentistry,
University of Leeds, Leeds, West Yorkshire, UK

Helen D. Rodd, BDS (Hons), PhD Department of Oral Health
and Development, School of Clinical Dentistry, University of Sheffield, Sheffield,
South Yorkshire, UK

W. Kim Seow, BDS, MDSc, PhD, DDSc Centre for Paediatric Dentistry,
School of Dentistry, University of Queensland, Brisbane,
QLD, Australia

Karin L. Weerheijm, PhD Paediatric Dentist KINDERTAND Zuid and member
Paediatric REsearch Project (PREP), Department of Cariology Endodontology
Pedodontology, Academic Centre for Dentistry (ACTA), Amsterdam,
The Netherlands

John Timothy Wright, DDS, MS Department of Pediatric Dentistry,
University of North Carolina, School of Dentistry, Chapel Hill, NC, USA

Dental Enamel Defects in the Primary Dentition: Prevalence and Etiology

1

W. Kim Seow

Abstract

The enamel of the primary dentition undergoes development from approximately the 13th week of gestation to around 3 years of age when the second primary molars erupt into the oral cavity. During this period, the developing primary dentition can be affected by many systemic and local environment insults that lead to changes in the quality and quantity of the enamel. The systemic influences that can cause abnormalities in the primary enamel range from pregnancy conditions such as pre-eclampsia to neonatal disruptions such as preterm births and postnatal infections such as rubella and chickenpox. The prevalence of enamel defects has been reported to range from approximately 30 % in the general population in USA, Britain, and Australia to over 70 % in preterm children and indigenous populations worldwide. The high prevalence of enamel hypoplasia reflects the vulnerability of developing teeth to environmental changes and suggests that complications of enamel defects, such as increased caries susceptibility, are common in the primary dentition.

The formation of enamel extends over a considerable period of time in the life of an individual. In the primary dentition, enamel formation commences at the tips of the incisors at approximately 15–19 weeks in utero and ends with the emergence of the second primary molars between 25 and 33 months of age [1]. During this long period of enamel development, many conditions can adversely affect the enamel-forming cells causing abnormalities to be produced. As enamel does not remodel, any aberrations occurring during formation may be permanently recorded on the surface as visible defects. Such developmental defects of enamel have major clinical significance. Some defects in the anterior teeth can affect aesthetics, cause severe tooth sensitivity, and impair masticatory function [2]. Importantly, enamel

W.K. Seow, BDS, MDSc, PhD, DDSc
Centre for Paediatric Dentistry, School of Dentistry, University of Queensland,
200 Turbot Street, Brisbane, QLD 4000, Australia
e-mail: k.seow@uq.edu.au

© Springer-Verlag Berlin Heidelberg 2015
B.K. Drummond, N. Kilpatrick (eds.), *Planning and Care for Children and Adolescents with Dental Enamel Defects: Etiology, Research and Contemporary Management*, DOI 10.1007/978-3-662-44800-7_1

defects in the primary dentition are now increasingly recognized as a major risk factor for early childhood caries (ECC) [3].

Presentations of Developmental Defects of Enamel (DDE)

The formation of enamel or amelogenesis begins during the late bell stage of tooth development when specialized enamel-forming cells, the ameloblasts, are differentiated from the inner enamel epithelium [4]. The initial stages of enamel formation are characterized by the secretion of specific proteins by the ameloblasts such as amelogenin and ameloblastin to form an enamel matrix which is later mineralized [5, 6]. After the laying down of the enamel matrix, the ameloblasts regulate the removal of water and proteins from the enamel matrix and promote the ingress of minerals [7]. The cellular and biochemical events that occur during amelogenesis are complex and can be adversely affected by genetic changes as well as by systemic and local environmental conditions.

Abnormalities that originate during the formation of enamel are commonly referred to as developmental defects of enamel (DDE) [8]. The presentation and severity of DDE are dependent on the stage of enamel development at the time of the insult, as well as the extent and duration of the adverse condition [9]. Quantitative deficiencies of DDE, which usually arise from disruptions of matrix formation, are known as enamel hypoplasia and may be expressed as pits, grooves, and thin or missing enamel [8]. In contrast, qualitative enamel deficiencies are usually associated with altered enamel mineralization and may be expressed as changes in the translucency or opacity of the enamel that may be diffuse or demarcated, and colored white, yellow, or brown [8]. Generally, it is thought that the more immature the stage of enamel formation, the more vulnerable to damage. Disturbances which occur during the secretory stages of enamel formation are generally thought to reduce the quantity of enamel formed, and this is usually expressed as enamel hypoplasia. In contrast, disturbances at the final stages are usually associated with altered mineralization of the enamel which manifests clinically as opacities. As the various primary teeth in a child's mouth may be at different stages of enamel formation at the time of an adverse condition, a spectrum of DDE, ranging from mild opacities to severe enamel hypoplasia, can result from a single insult.

As DDE are permanent records of enamel changes, the location of a defect on the enamel surface can suggest the timing of the events that disrupted enamel formation. Although exact timing is often difficult to identify, knowledge of the chronology of development of the primary tooth crowns may be useful in estimating the approximate times of the insults (Table 1.1). Table 1.1 shows that the primary teeth usually commence mineralization in utero, starting with primary central incisors at approximately 15–19 weeks, canines at 16–22 weeks, first molars at 19–22 weeks, and second molars at 20–22 weeks [1]. At birth, the amount of enamel formed is approximately three-quarters, two-thirds, and one-third of the primary central incisor, lateral incisor, and canine crowns respectively. In addition, at birth, the first molar cusps are usually formed, but not coalesced, and the second molar cusp tips are commencing initial mineralization. Table 1.1 also shows that crown formation is

Table 1.1 Chronology of tooth crown formation of the primary dentition

Primary tooth	Tooth formation commences	Amount of crown formed at birth	Crown completed
Incisors	15–19 weeks in utero	Central incisors: three-quarters	1.5–3 months
		Lateral incisors: two-thirds	
First molar	16–22 weeks in utero	Cusps formed, not coalesced	5.5–6 months
Canine	19–22 weeks in utero	One-third of cusp	9–10 months
Second molar	20–22 weeks in utero	Tips of cusps	10–11 months

Reprinted from Sunderland et al. [1]. With permission from Elsevier

complete in the primary incisors by 3 months, the first molars by 6 months, the canines by 10 months, and the second primary molars by 12 months. After complete crown formation, the newly formed enamel undergoes a process of maturation and hardening that continues post-eruption [4].

The enamel formed prenatally may be demarcated from that formed postnatally by an area of altered enamel known as the neonatal line. This band of abnormal enamel has a disorganized prism alignment and contains more organic material compared to the adjacent enamel [10]. As the entire primary dentition commences calcification before birth, the neonatal line is usually present in all primary teeth [11]. It may widen to a clinically visible area of abnormal enamel if a child experiences adverse neonatal conditions such as fetal distress and difficult birth delivery. Many DDE associated with perinatal illnesses are thus located at the neonatal line.

Prevalence

Several indices have been utilized to record DDE, the most popular being a descriptive index, the Developmental Defects of Enamel (DDE) index which does not attempt to identify the etiology [8]. There have been several modifications of this index, including simplified versions that can be applied for screening purposes. Many authors use the simplified modifications of the index to record DDE in the primary dentition for practical reasons [8]. Variations in prevalence of DDE reported in different populations are likely to be the result of differing criteria being used to define enamel defects. In addition, there are population variations resulting from differences in general health, and background fluoride exposure levels may also contribute to differences in the reported prevalence of DDE. Furthermore, in many studies, the recording of DDE in primary teeth several years post-eruption may be complicated by difficulties in diagnosing DDE once the lesions have become carious or have been restored [12]. Finally, differing field conditions during examination for DDE, such as variations in lighting and whether the teeth are dried prior to recording of the defects, may also contribute to differences in reported prevalence.

As there are few high-quality studies, the true prevalence of DDE in the primary dentition is unclear. Most prevalence studies on the primary dentition have been based on convenient samples from the general or special population groups such as medically compromised children. Table 1.2 lists selected reports of prevalence of DDE in the primary dentition published since 1996. There are significant variations

Table 1.2 Prevalence of DDE in the primary dentition by country

Authors	Year	Country	Prevalence
Li et al. [13]	1995	China	22 %
Slayton et al. [14]	2001	USA	33 %
Montero et al. [15]	2003	USA	49 %
Lunardelli and Peres [16]	2005	Brazil	24 %
Chaves et al. [17]	2007	Brazil	44 %
Elfink et al. [18]	2008	Holland	5 % (primary 2nd molars only)
Hong et al. [19]	2009	USA	4 % (primary molars only)
Casanova-Rosado et al. [20]	2011	Mexico	10 %
Seow et al. [21]	2011	Australia	25 %
Correa-Faria et al. [22]	2013	Brazil	30 %
Masumo et al. [23]	2013	Tanzania	33 %
Ghanim et al. [24]	2013	Iraq	7 % (primary 2nd molars only)

in prevalence rates among different countries and population groups. A Chinese study showed that primary teeth with defective enamel were seen in 24 % of children, with opacities contributing 2 % and enamel hypoplasia 22 % [13]. In the USA, the study of Slayton and co-workers [14] reported a total prevalence of DDE in the primary dentition of 33 %, with 6 % of healthy children having at least one tooth with enamel hypoplasia and 27 % having enamel opacities [14]. In another USA study, Montero and co-workers reported an overall prevalence of DDE in the primary dentition of 49 % [15], while in Mexico, a DDE prevalence of only 10 % was found [20]. In Australia, the prevalence of DDE was reported to be 25 % in a primary school cohort [21], compared with a rate of approximately 24–44 % in Brazil [16, 17, 22]. In Holland, the prevalence of hypomineralized second primary molars was reported at 5 % and 4 % at the child and tooth level, respectively, with the majority of DDE being demarcated opacities [18]. More recently, a study in Iraq reported that 7 % of children had hypomineralization defects in at least one second primary molar [24]. In Tanzania, the prevalence of enamel defects was 33 %, with diffuse opacities constituting the most common defects (23 %), followed by hypoplasia (8 %) and demarcated opacities (5 %). In that study, the most frequently affected teeth were the primary central incisors (approximately 30 %), whereas lower central incisors (4–5 %) were least frequently affected [23]. Many indigenous communities, for example, in Australia, Canada, and the USA are reported to have higher rates of DDE, probably due to increased risks for poorer general health compared to other communities [25].

Distribution

In a study of over 3,200 primary teeth, 5 % of primary teeth had some form of DDE, and the most prevalent defects were found, in descending order, in the mandibular second molar, maxillary second molar, mandibular canine, mandibular first molar, maxillary first molar, maxillary lateral and central incisors, and maxillary canine

[21]. Only a very small percentage of the mandibular central and lateral incisors exhibited DDE, and these were mainly enamel opacities [21]. In addition, the most common type of DDE found in the primary dentition was the demarcated opacity, followed, in turn, by diffuse opacity and enamel hypoplasia. In another study, the maxillary primary central and lateral incisors were affected by enamel hypoplasia at the highest frequencies (41 % and 39 %), followed by the maxillary canines (26 %), maxillary first molars (22 %), and mandibular first molars (19 %) [13].

Etiology

Table 1.3 shows the plethora of conditions that have been associated with DDE in primary teeth. Hereditary conditions such as amelogenesis imperfecta are caused by abnormalities in genes involved in enamel formation [26]. Other forms of DDE that may be inherited include those that are inherited as familial disorders or dysmorphic syndromes that show enamel defects [27]. Acquired systemic conditions that can cause DDE may be encountered perinatally, neonatally, or postnatally and include conditions such as birth trauma, metabolic conditions, and infections. Adverse conditions experienced by the mother during pregnancy that may cause DDE in the child include severe maternal vitamin D deficiency [28] and infection with syphilis [29]. Local factors impacting on the oral cavity, such as trauma and radiation, can also cause many DDE in the primary dentition. However, evidence

Table 1.3 Etiology of developmental dental defects in the primary dentition

Generalized defects
I. Inherited
Amelogenesis imperfecta
Generalized inherited disorder or syndrome with enamel defect
II. Acquired systemic condition perinatally, neonatally, or postnatally
Maternal conditions during pregnancy, e.g., cytomegalovirus infection, vitamin D deficiency
Birth trauma
Preterm birth
Isolated cleft lip and palate
Nutritional deficiencies
Renal and liver conditions, e.g., renal failure, biliary atresia
Celiac disease
Endocrine, e.g., hypocalcemia, hypoglycemia
Infections from bacteria, viruses and fungi
Chemicals and toxins
Other systemic conditions
Localized factors
I. Trauma, e.g., laryngoscopy
II. Radiation, e.g., cancer treatment
III. Local infection

for the associations between many of the acquired systemic conditions and DDE are based mainly on clinical studies and case reports. There are only a few instances such as the use of tetracyclines where direct causal links have been demonstrated between an individual adverse condition and enamel changes in primary teeth [30].

Systemic Factors

Hereditary Conditions

Amelogenesis Imperfecta

Amelogenesis imperfecta is a genetic condition in which both dentitions are characterized by enamel defects and will be discussed in detail in Chap. 5.

Generalized Inherited Disorder or Syndrome with DDE

There are several hereditary syndromes that affect the development of enamel in the primary and permanent dentitions (see Chap. 4). In inherited dermatological syndromes involving the skin, hair, and nails e.g. ectodermal dysplasia, epidermolysis bullosa, and tuberous sclerosis, both primary and permanent dentitions usually show generalized DDE [2]. In addition, hereditary conditions associated with defects in mineralization pathways that involve the parathyroid glands and vitamin D metabolism often show abnormalities of enamel development. The hypoparathyroidism featured in the velocardiofacial syndrome is thought to be associated with DDE in the primary dentition. The links between hypoparathyroidism and enamel defects are also encountered in rare congenital conditions such as the autoimmune polyendocrinopathy-candidiasis-ectodermal dystrophy syndrome [31]. In the inherited types of rickets, e.g., vitamin D-resistant rickets, generalized enamel hypoplasia often results from chronic hypocalcemia/hypophosphatemia present in this condition [32].

Acquired Systemic Conditions

Numerous acquired conditions have been associated with DDE in the primary dentition. Such conditions may be systemic or local and may be timed to the antenatal, perinatal, or postnatal periods of development. Prenatal factors that have been associated with DDE in the primary dentition include failure to access antenatal care, increased maternal weight gain during pregnancy, pre-eclampsia and maternal smoking [33]. Maternal vitamin D deficiency during pregnancy that is associated with hyperparathyroidism has also been associated with enamel defects [28].

Birth Trauma and Adverse Perinatal Conditions

During the time of birth, adverse factors that have been reported to cause DDE include birth trauma, hypoglycemia, hypocalcemia and neonatal tetany. Many children with cerebral palsy caused by fetal distress and children with toxic levels of

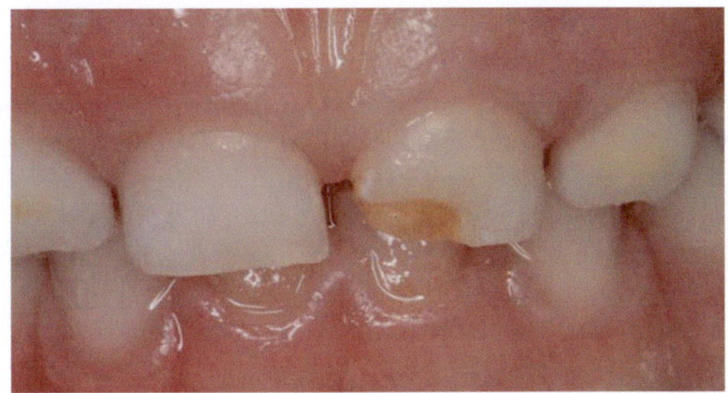

Fig. 1.1 The maxillary primary left central incisor from a premature born child shows severe enamel hypoplasia that is most likely caused by traumatic intubation

bilirubin (hyperbilirubinemia) associated with systemic conditions such congenital bile duct and liver disease have DDE in the primary dentition. In these children it is thought that the damage sustained by the ameloblasts reflects the systemic disturbances caused by these conditions [34, 35].

Premature Birth

The DDE found in prematurely born children may be associated with neonatal complications of birth prematurity such as respiratory, cardiovascular, gastrointestinal and renal abnormalities, intracranial hemorrhage, hyperbilirubinemia and/or anemia. Deficient gastrointestinal absorption and inadequate supplies of calcium and phosphorus have also been associated with DDE in the primary teeth of prematurely born children [36]. Children who are born premature with low birth weight have been reported to show a higher prevalence of DDE compared to children born full term with normal birth weight. In children with birth weights less than 1,500 g and between 1,500 and 2,500 g, the prevalences were found to be 62 and 27 %, respectively, compared with only 13 % in children with normal birth weight [37]. In addition, in utero insults associated with small-for-gestational status have been recently suggested as an important cause of enamel hypomineralization/hypoplasia in primary teeth of very low birth weight children [38].

Local trauma may occur from laryngoscopy and endotracheal intubation which are often required in prematurely born children during management of respiratory distress. This can disrupt development of teeth [39]. In a preterm child, due to the lack of fulcrum support from an extremely small mandible, the laryngoscope is often placed on the anterior maxillary alveolus during intubation. This may result in inadvertent pressure being exerted on the developing primary maxillary incisor teeth. In severe cases, crown distortions, dilacerations and enamel hypoplasia/hypomineralization can result from such trauma from the laryngoscope. As the pressure from the laryngoscope is usually exerted on the left side, the most common teeth affected from laryngoscope trauma are the maxillary left incisor teeth. Figure 1.1 shows a maxillary primary left central incisor with severe enamel hypoplasia in a prematurely born child caused by traumatic intubation during the neonatal period.

Isolated Cleft Lip and Palate

Children with isolated cleft lip and palate have a higher DDE prevalence compared to normal children, most likely due to the local tissue disruption caused by the clefting anomaly on enamel formation. DDE in the primary maxillary central incisors has been reported in 43 % of children with unilateral cleft lip, with the defects occurring mainly on the cleft side [40]. In another study of 4-year-old children with cleft lip and palate, 56 % had enamel defects which were mostly opacities [41].

Malnutrition and Nutritional Deficiencies

Postnatal factors occurring in children under the age of 12 months that may cause DDE in the primary dentition include malnutrition [42] and nutritional deficiencies particularly intake deficiency and gut malabsorption of vitamins A, C and D; calcium; and phosphorous [43]. In addition, extended breastfeeding without solid supplementation can cause suboptimal nutrition that may be associated with DDE in young children [33].

Liver and Renal Conditions

As the liver and kidneys are involved in the activation of vitamin D and the calcification of bone and teeth, children with liver and renal diseases may be at increased risk of DDE. In one study over 19 % of children with chronic kidney failure were shown to have DDE in the primary teeth compared to only 3 % of otherwise unaffected controls [44]. In congenital liver diseases, high levels of circulating bilirubin cause disruption of ameloblast function which can lead to formation of defects in the developing enamel (Fig. 1.2) [45].

Celiac Disease and Gastrointestinal Malabsorption

Children with celiac disease may have malabsorption and mineral deficiencies associated with gut enteropathy. Celiac disease is caused by inflammation of the bowel resulting from gliadins (gluten proteins) found in wheat and barley triggering the formation of antibodies which react with the small-bowel tissue. Atrophy of the intestinal villus results from the inflammation, and absorption of nutrients such as vitamin D, calcium and phosphorus from the small bowel is affected [46]. As a result of the malabsorption, children with celiac disease are at high risk for DDE [47, 48]. Scanning electron microscopic studies have shown that the enamel of children with celiac disease is less mineralized and more irregular compared to normal teeth [49]. All permanent teeth in children with celiac disease are at risk however in the primary dentition; the molars are more likely to be affected as they undergo a significant part of their mineralization after the introduction of gluten into the diet [50].

Infections

Serious systemic infections during pregnancy and in infancy have been shown to be associated with DDE in the primary dentition. Potential mechanisms include the infective microorganisms damaging the ameloblasts directly or altering their cellular function indirectly through their metabolic products. High temperatures in young

Fig. 1.2 (**a**) The restored primary dentition of a child with a history of hyperbilirubinemia from birth. (**b**) Note the attempt to improve the aesthetics of the upper incisors by placement of labial composite resin veneers (Courtesy of Professor B Drummond)

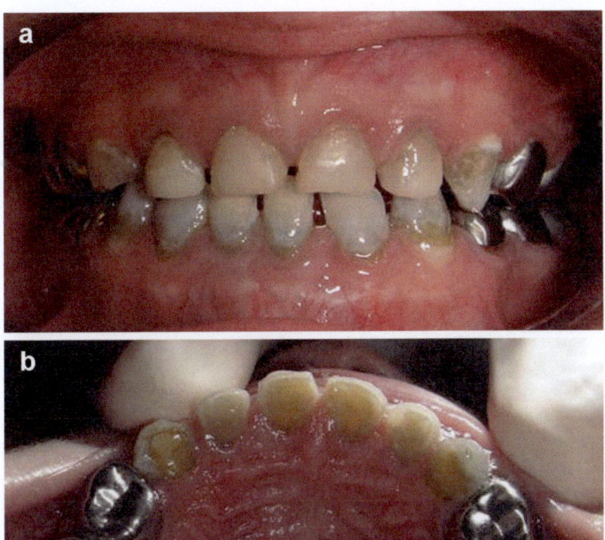

children associated with urinary tract infections, otitis media and respiratory tract diseases may also affect ameloblast function resulting in defects of enamel [51]. Bacterial infections including congenital syphilis and meningococcal disease have also been shown to cause DDE in the primary dentition [52]. Viral infections, in either the mother during pregnancy or the infant postnatally such as chickenpox, rubella, measles, mumps and cytomegalovirus are also well known to be associated with DDE [29]. Figure 1.3 shows a mandibular primary second molar with enamel hypoplasia that is associated with a previous severe viral infection that occurred at approximately 12 months of age.

Chemicals and Toxins

Ameloblasts are also highly sensitive to many chemicals and drugs, and DDE have been reported to result from exposure to agents such as fluoride and some antibiotics or cytotoxic drugs such as those used in chemotherapy. High doses of fluoride have been shown to cause hypoplasia and enamel opacities in animal models [53]. However prolonged, inadvertent or deliberate ingestion of fluoride toothpaste by 2- to 3-year-olds can only cause hypomineralization of developing permanent enamel as mineralization of the primary teeth is already completed by this age [54]. Ingestion of fluoride by the mother during pregnancy is not linked to DDE as little fluoride crosses the placental barrier. Mild diffuse opacities in the primary dentition have been reported following exposure to high levels of fluoride in water [55]. One

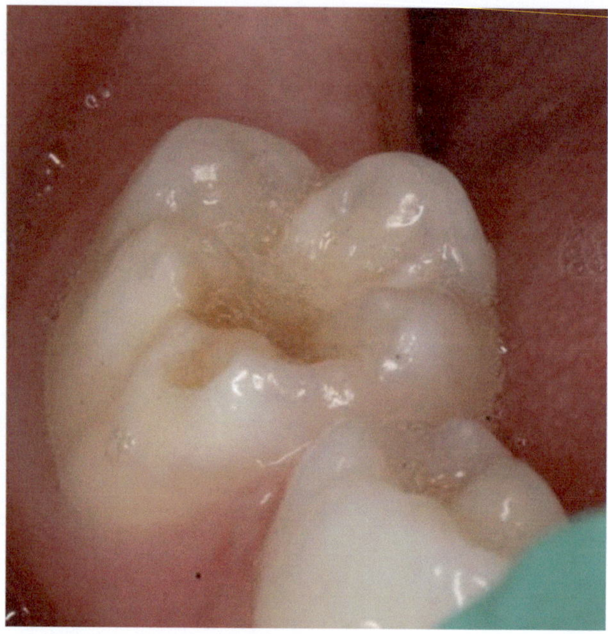

Fig. 1.3 A mandibular primary second molar showing enamel hypoplasia that is associated with a severe viral infection at approximately 12 months of age

study has suggested that children ingesting fluoride supplements from 6 to 9 months of age have an increased risk for fluorosis in the primary second molars [56].

High levels of lead from environmental exposures, accidental or pica ingestion have been shown to cause DDE in the primary dentition [57]. Tetracyclines are also well known to cause dental discolorations and enamel hypoplasia [30]. Although most previous reports of tetracycline staining are of permanent teeth, any primary teeth developing during the time of tetracycline intake could also theoretically be affected.

Other Systemic Conditions

Multiple birth children are at increased risk for DDE. In a controlled twin study, 21 and 22 % of monozygotic and dizygotic twins had DDE, compared to only 15 % in singleton children [58]. To date, minimal genetic influence has been found for DDE from twin studies and the higher prevalence of DDE in twins is likely to be associated with the greater rate of neonatal complications such as premature births experienced by multiple birth children.

Although many clinical conditions have been identified as suggested causes of DDE, it is also possible that the defects result from undiagnosed or subclinical conditions where there is damage to the ameloblasts without obvious clinical symptoms in the children. For example, in a study of babies who died of sudden infant death syndrome (a condition of unknown causes), there was good correlation between identified enamel defects in the primary teeth and the antemortem history and the autopsy findings [59].

Local Factors Causing DDE

Local insults such as trauma involve only the teeth in the immediate area of damage in contrast to systemic factors which usually affect all developing teeth. For example, local trauma exerted through the thin buccal cortical bone is thought to be the cause of demarcated opacities commonly observed on the labial surfaces of primary canines [60]. The reason for the primary canines being at highest risk for DDE is the fact that the cortical buccal bone overlying the canines is thin, and the developing tooth buds situated beneath the cortical bone are easily traumatized by external pressure from accidents, falls or blows etc. Developing teeth exposed to radiation for treatment of tumors or leukemia are also known to be at risk for a range of developmental defects including DDE [61].

In conclusion, the high prevalence of enamel defects that is reported in the primary dentitions of some children reflects the vulnerability of these developing teeth to environmental changes during gestation and in the immediate postnatal period. Given the reported complications associated with DDE, such as increased caries susceptibility, it is important that these defects are identified in young children as early as possible so that appropriately targeted prevention can be established.

References

 1. Sunderland EP, Smith CJ, Sunderland R. A histological study of the chronology of initial mineralization in the human deciduous dentition. Arch Oral Biol. 1987;32(3):167–74.
 2. Salanitri S, Seow WK. Developmental enamel defects in the primary dentition: aetiology and clinical management. Aust Dent J. 2013;58(2):133–40.
 3. Caufield PW, Li Y, Bromage TG. Hypoplasia-associated severe early childhood caries – a proposed definition. J Dent Res. 2013;91:544–50.
 4. Nanci A. Enamel: composition, formation, and structure. In: Nanci A, editor. Ten Cate's oral histology development, structure, and function. St. Louis: Mosby; 2008. p. 141–90.
 5. Simmer JP, Fincham AG. Molecular mechanisms of dental enamel formation. Crit Rev Oral Biol Med. 1995;6(2):84–108.
 6. Gibson C. The amelogenin proteins and enamel development in humans and mice. J Oral Biosci. 2011;53:248–56.
 7. Fukae M. Enamel formation – biochemical aspects. J Oral Biosci. 2009;51(1):46–60.
 8. Clarkson J, O'Mullane DM. A modified DDE index for use in epidemiological studies of enamel defects. J Dent Res. 1989;68:445–50.
 9. Seow WK. Developmental defects of enamel and dentine: challenges for basic science research and clinical management. Aust Dent J. 2014;59(1 Suppl):1–12.
10. Sabel N, Johansson C, Kühnisch J, Robertson A, Steiniger F, Norén JG, et al. Neonatal lines in the enamel of primary teeth – a morphological and scanning electron microscopic investigation. Arch Oral Biol. 2008;53(10):954–63.
11. Mahoney P. Human deciduous mandibular molar incremental enamel development. Am J Phys Anthropol. 2011;144(2):204–14.
12. Seow WK. Clinical diagnosis of enamel defects: pitfalls and practical guidelines. Int Dent J. 1997;47(3):173–82.
13. Li Y, Navia JM, Bian JH. Prevalence and distribution of developmental enamel defects in primary dentition of Chinese children 3–5 years old. Community Dent Oral Epidemiol. 1995;23(2):72–9.

14. Slayton R, Warren J, Kanellis M, Levy S, Islam M. Prevalence of enamel hypoplasia and isolated opacities in the primary dentition. Pediatr Dent. 2001;23:32–6.
15. Montero MJ, Douglass JM, Mathieu G. Prevalence of dental caries and enamel defects in Connecticut head start children. Pediatr Dent. 2003;25:235–9.
16. Lunardelli S, Peres M. Prevalence and distribution of developmental enamel defects in the primary dentition of pre-school children. Braz Oral Res. 2005;19:144–9.
17. Chaves AMB, Rosenblatt A, Oliveira OFB. Enamel defects and its relation to life course events in primary dentition of Brazilian children: a longitudinal study. Community Dent Health. 2007;24:31–6.
18. Elfrink MEC, Schuller AA, Weerheijm KL, Veerkamp JSJ. Hypomineralized second primary molars: prevalence data in Dutch 5-year-olds. Caries Res. 2008;42(4):282–5.
19. Hong L, Levy SM, Warren JJ, Bergus GR, Dawson DV, Wefel JS, et al. Association between enamel hypoplasia and dental caries in primary second molars: a cohort study. Caries Res. 2009;43:345–53.
20. Casanova-Rosado AJ, Medina-Solıs CE, Casanova-Rosado JF. Association between developmental enamel defects in the primary and permanent dentitions. Eur J Paediatr Dent. 2011;12:155–8.
21. Seow WK, Ford D, Kazoullis S, Newman B, Holcombe T. Comparison of enamel defects in the primary and permanent dentitions of children from a low-fluoride district in Australia. Pediatr Dent. 2011;33:207–12.
22. Correa-Faria P, Martins-Junior PA, Vieira-Andrade RG, Oliveira-Ferreira F, Marques LS, Ramos-Jorge ML. Developmental defects of enamel in primary teeth: prevalence and associated factors. Int J Paediatr Dent. 2012;23:173–9.
23. Masumo R, Bardsen A, Astrom A. Developmental defects of enamel in primary teeth and association with early life course events: a study of 6–36 month old children in Manyara, Tanzania. BMC Oral Health. 2013;13(1):21.
24. Ghanim A, Manton D, Marino R, Morgan M, Bailey D. Prevalence of demarcated hypomineralisation defects in second primary molars in Iraqi children. Int J Paediatr Dent. 2013;23(1):48–55.
25. Pascoe L, Seow WK. Enamel hypoplasia and dental caries in Australian aboriginal children: prevalence and correlation between the two diseases. Pediatr Dent. 1994;16(3):193–9.
26. Wright TC, Hart PS, Michalec MD, Seow WK, Hart TC. Identification of a novel enamelin mutation (g.8344delG) in a family with amelogenesis imperfecta. Arch Oral Biol. 2003;48:589–96.
27. Seow WK. Trichodentoosseous (TDO) syndrome: case report and literature review. Pediatr Dent. 1993;15(5):355–61.
28. Purvis RJ, MacKay GS, Barrie WJM. Enamel hypoplasia of the teeth associated with neonatal tetany: a manifestation of maternal vitamin D deficiency. Lancet. 1973;2(7833):811–4.
29. Jaskoll T, Abichaker G, Htet K. Cytomegalovirus induces stage-dependent enamel defects and misexpression of amelogenin, enamelin and dentin sialophosphoprotein in developing mouse molars. Cells Tissue Organs. 2010;192:221–39.
30. Witkop Jr CJ, Wolf RO. Hypoplasia and intrinsic staining of enamel following tetracycline therapy. JAMA. 1963;185(13):1008–11.
31. Pavlič A, Waltimo-Sirén J. Clinical and microstructural aberrations of enamel of deciduous and permanent teeth in patients with autoimmune polyendocrinopathy–candidiasis–ectodermal dystrophy. Arch Oral Biol. 2009;54(7):658–65.
32. Goodman JR, Gelbier MJ, Bennett JH, Winter GB. Dental problems associated with hypophosphataemic vitamin D resistant rickets. Int J Paediatr Dent. 1998;8:19–28.
33. Needleman HL, Allred E, Bellinger D, Leviton A, Rabinowitz M, Iverson K. Antecedents and correlates of hypoplastic enamel defects of primary incisors. Pediatr Dent. 1992;14(3):158–66.
34. Bhat M, Nelson KB, Cummins SK, Grether JK. Prevalence of developmental enamel defects in children with cerebral palsy. J Oral Pathol Med. 1992;21(6):241–4.

35. Lin X, Wu W, Zhang C, Lo EC, Chu CH, Dissanayaka WL. Prevalence and distribution of developmental enamel defects in children with cerebral palsy in Beijing, China. Int J Paediatr Dent. 2011;21(1):23–8.
36. Seow W, Masel JP, Weir C, Tudehope DI. Mineral deficiency in the pathogenesis of enamel hypoplasia in prematurely born, very low birthweight children. Pediatr Dent. 1989; 11(4):297–302.
37. Seow WK, Humphrys C, Tudehope DI. Increased prevalence of developmental dental defects in low-birth-weight children: a controlled study. Pediatr Dent. 1987;9:221–5.
38. Nelson S, Albert JM, Geng C, Curtan S, Lang K, Miadich S, et al. Increased enamel hypoplasia and very low birthweight infants. J Dent Res. 2013;92(9):788–94.
39. Seow WK, Brown JP, Tudehope DI, O'Callaghan M. Developmental defects in the primary dentition of low birth-weight infants: adverse effects of laryngoscopy and prolonged endotracheal intubation. Pediatr Dent. 1984;6:28–31.
40. Gomes AC, Neves LT, Gomide MR. Enamel defects in maxillary central incisors of infants with unilateral cleft lip. Cleft Palate Craniofac J. 2009;46(4):420–4.
41. Chapple JR, Nunn JH. The oral health of children with clefts of the lip, palate, or both. Cleft Palate Craniofac J. 2001;38(5):525–8.
42. Rugg-Gunn AJ, Al-Mohammadi SM, Butler TJ. Malnutrition and developmental defects of enamel in 2- to 6-year-old Saudi boys. Caries Res. 1998;32(3):181–92.
43. Takaoka LAMV, Goulart AL, Kopelman BI, Weiler RME. Enamel defects in the complete primary dentition of children born at term and preterm. Pediatr Dent. 2011;33(2):171–6.
44. Koch MJ, Bührer R, Pioch T, Schärer K. Enamel hypoplasia of primary teeth in chronic renal failure. Pediatr Nephrol. 1999;13(1):68–72.
45. Seow W, Shepherd R, Ong T. Oral changes associated with end-stage liver disease and liver transplantation: implications for dental management. ASDC J Dent Child. 1991; 58(6):474–80.
46. Di Sabatino A, Corazza G. Coeliac disease. Lancet. 2009;373(9673):1480–93.
47. Majorana A, Bardellini E, Ravelli A, Plebani A, Polimeni A, Campus G. Implications of gluten exposure period, CD clinical forms, and HLA typing in the association between celiac disease and dental enamel defects in children. A case–control study. Int J Paediatr Dent. 2010;20(2):119–24.
48. Páez EO, Lafuente PJ, García PB, Lozano JM, Calvo JCL. Prevalence of dental enamel defects in celiac patients with deciduous dentition: a pilot study. Oral Surg. 2008;106(1):898–902.
49. Bossu M, Bartoli A, Orsini G, Luppino E, Polimeni A. Enamel hypoplasia in coeliac children: a potential clinical marker of early diagnosis. Eur J Paediatr Dent. 2007;8(1):31–7.
50. Ortega Paez E, Junco Lafuente P, Baca Garcia P, Maldonado Lozano J, Llodra Calvo JC. Prevalence of dental enamel defects in celiac patients with deciduous dentition: a pilot study. Oral Surg Oral Med Oral Pathol Oral Radiol Endod. 2008;106(1):74–8.
51. Ford D, Seow WK, Kazoullis S, Holcombe T, Newman B. A controlled study of risk factors for enamel hypoplasia in the permanent dentition. Pediatr Dent. 2009;31(5):382–8.
52. Patterson MDH. Syphilis (*Treponema pallidum*). In: Kliegman RM, Behrman RE, Jenson HB, Stanton BF, editors. Nelson textbook of pediatrics. Philadelphia: Saunders Elsevier; 2011.
53. Suckling GW, Purdell-Lewis D. Macroscopic appearance, microhardness and microradiographic characteristics of experimentally produced fluorotic lesions in sheep enamel. Caries Res. 1982;16(3):227–34.
54. Browne D, Whelton H, O'Mullane DM. Fluoride metabolism and fluorosis. J Dent. 2005;33(3):177–86.
55. Weeks KJ, Milsom KM, Lennon MA. Enamel defects in 4- to 5-year-old children in fluoridated and non-fluoridated parts of Cheshire, UK. Caries Res. 1993;27(4):317–20.
56. Levy SM, Hillis SL, Warren JJ, Broffitt BA, Mahbubul Islam AKM, Wefel JS, et al. Primary tooth fluorosis and fluoride intake during the first year of life. Community Dent Oral Epidemiol. 2002;30(4):286–95.

57. Gerlach RF, Cury JA, Krug FJ, Line SRP. Effect of lead on dental enamel formation. Toxicology. 2002;175(1–3):27–34.
58. Taji S, Seow WK, Townsend GC, Holcombe T. Enamel hypoplasia in the primary dentition of monozygotic and dizygotic twins compared with singleton controls. Int J Paediatr Dent. 2011;21(3):175–84.
59. Teivens A, Mörnstad H, Norén JG, Gidlund E. Enamel incremental lines as recorders for disease in infancy and their relation to the diagnosis of SIDS. Forensic Sci Int. 1996; 81(2–3):175–83.
60. Lukacs JR. Localized enamel hypoplasia of human deciduous canine teeth: prevalence and pattern of expression in rural Pakistan. Hum Biol. 1991;63:513–22.
61. Weyman J. The effect of irradiation on developing teeth. Oral Surg Oral Med Oral Pathol. 1968;25(4):623–9.

Enamel Defects in the Permanent Dentition: Prevalence and Etiology

2

Robert P. Anthonappa and Nigel M. King

Abstract

The prevalence of developmental defects of enamel (DDE) in the permanent dentition in developed countries has been reported to be in the range of 9–68 % and with no gender predilection. Several etiological factors have been implicated as being responsible for DDE in the permanent teeth. Although local, systemic, genetic or environmental factors have been attributed to DDE frequently they are likely to be multifactorial in nature. These factors are discussed in relation to the timing of enamel development with consideration of the evidence, or lack thereof, for the association between the putative etiological factors and the nature of the subsequent abnormalities.

Introduction

The first permanent tooth to begin calcification is the first molar. This occurs around the time of birth, while the anterior teeth commence calcification between 4 and 6 months of age in a sequential order from the central incisor to the canine. The maxillary lateral incisor is the exception as calcification of this tooth occurs around 10–12 months of age [1]. At around 6 years of age, the first permanent molar tooth begins to erupt into the oral cavity and by the age of 14 years, most children have all of their permanent teeth erupted except for their third molars (Table 2.1). Many factors have been implicated in the etiology of developmental defects of enamel (DDE) in permanent teeth. This chapter discusses these factors in relation to the timing of

R.P. Anthonappa, BDS, MDS, PhD • N.M. King, BDS Hons MSc Hons, PhD (✉)
Department of Paediatric Dentistry, School of Dentistry, Faculty of Medicine, Dentistry and Health Sciences, University of Western Australia, 17 Monash Avenue, Nedlands, Perth, WA 6009, Australia
e-mail: robert.anthonappa@uwa.edu.au;
nigel.king@uwa.edu.au, profnigelking@mac.com

© Springer-Verlag Berlin Heidelberg 2015
B.K. Drummond, N. Kilpatrick (eds.), *Planning and Care for Children and Adolescents with Dental Enamel Defects: Etiology, Research and Contemporary Management*, DOI 10.1007/978-3-662-44800-7_2

Table 2.1 The calcification and eruption dates of permanent teeth

Permanent tooth type	Calcification begins at	Crown formation completes at	Eruption[a]	
			Maxillary	Mandibular
Central incisor	3–4 mo	4–5 y	7–8 y	6–7 y
Lateral incisor	Maxilla: 10–12 mo	4–5 y	8–9 y	7–8 y
	Mandible: 3–4 mo	4–5 y		
Canine	4–5 mo	6–7 y	11–12 y	9–11 y
First premolar	18–24 mo	5–6 y	10–11 y	10–12 y
Second premolar	24–30 mo	6–7 y	10–12 y	11–13 y
First molar	Birth	30–36 mo	5.5–7 y	5.5–7 y
Second molar	30–36 mo	7–8 y	12–14 y	12–14 y
Third molar	Maxilla: 7–9 y		>16 y	>16 y
	Mandible: 8–10 y			

mo months, *y* year
[a]It is noteworthy that the sequence is not simply in rank order

enamel development and considers the evidence, or lack thereof, for the association between the etiological factors and the nature of the subsequent abnormalities.

Prevalence of DDE in the Permanent Dentition

Mouth and tooth prevalence are the most commonly used systems to report the prevalence data for DDE. Mouth prevalence is determined by the inclusion of any individual who has been found to have at least one tooth affected by the condition, while tooth prevalence illustrates the percentage of teeth affected per person. Mouth prevalence figures reflect the extent of the distribution of enamel defects in a population group because individuals who are mildly and severely affected are grouped together. Tooth prevalence indicates the proportion of teeth affected and hence reflects the severity of the condition [2].

Table 2.2 summarizes the prevalence of DDE in the permanent dentition as reported in the literature. Wide variations exist in the literature because of the use of various terminologies and the different diagnostic criteria employed to describe the enamel defects in the permanent dentition [21, 22, 24, 26]. Nevertheless, the majority of reports have failed to demonstrate any difference in the prevalence of enamel defects between girls and boys [12, 27]. Furthermore, for all types of enamel defects, the published mouth prevalence in the permanent dentition ranges from 9.8 % to 93 % [8, 26], while tooth prevalence figures range from 2.2 % to 21.6 % [26, 28].

Etiology of DDE in the Permanent Dentition

Enamel morphogenesis is a continuous, complex process that starts with the secretion of enamel matrix proteins followed by mineralization and finally maturation. This process has been shown to start at the cusps on the molars and the incisal part

Table 2.2 The prevalence figures, reported in the literature, for any type developmental defects of enamel in the permanent dentition of healthy children

Author	Year	Country	F level (ppm)	Age (years)	Prevalence % Mouth	Tooth
Suckling et al. [3]	1985	New Zealand	1.0	12	56.6	18.8
Dooland and Wylie [4]	1989	Australia	1.0	8–9	–	25.5
			0			15.6
Dummer et al. [5]	1990	UK	<0.1	15–16	50.1	5.71
					26.2	11.8
Nunn et al. [6]	1992	UK	<0.2	15	64.1	38.7
					–	57.5
			1.0		78.9	59
					–	83.9
			1.0–1.3		83.9	66.2
					–	81.5
Fyffe et al. [7]	1996	UK	–	13–14	48.7	–
Rugg-Gunn et al. [8]	1997	Saudi Arabia	0.25	14	75	–
			0.80		82	–
			2.71		93	–
Hiller et al. [9]	1998	Germany	<0.02	8–10	39.9	
Dini et al. [10]	2000	Brazil	0.7	9–10	26.1	–
Jalevik et al. [11]	2001	Sweden	Low	7–8	33.3	–
Zagdwon et al. [12]	2002	UK	<0.1	7	14.5	7.2
Ekanayake and van der Hoek [13]	2003	Sri Lanka	<0.3	14	29	–
			0.3–0.5		35	
			0.5–0.7		43	–
			>0.7		57	–
Cochran et al. [14]	2004	Finland	<0.01	8	59	–
		Greece	<0.01		43	–
		Iceland	0.05		54	–
		Portugal	0.08		49	–
		UK	<0.1		48	–
		The Netherlands	0.13		70	–
		Ireland	1.0		69	–
Mackay and Thomson [15]	2005	New Zealand	–	9–10	51.6	–
Balmer et al. [16]	2005	UK	<0.1	8–16	–	27.3
		Australia	0.9–1.1			51.6
Wong et al. [17]	2006	Hong Kong	1.0 (1983)	12	92.1	–
			0.7 (1991)		55.8	–
			0.5 (2001)		35.2	–
Hoffmann et al. [18]	2007	Brazil	–	12	46.4	–
Muratbegovic et al. [19]	2008	Bosnia and Herzegovina	<0.1	12	32.8	–
Arrow [20]	2008	Australia	0.8	7	22	–
Kanagaratnam et al. [21]	2009	New Zealand	–	9	35[a]	–

(continued)

Table 2.2 (continued)

Author	Year	Country	F level (ppm)	Age (years)	Prevalence %	
					Mouth	Tooth
Seow et al. [22]	2011	Australia	0.1	13.5[b]	58	–
Casanova-Rosado et al. [23]	2011	Mexico	–	6–12	7.5	–
Robles et al. [24]	2013	Spain	0.07	3–12	52	8.3
Vargas-Ferreira et al. [25]	2014	Brazil	–	8–12	64	–

[a]Both fluoridated and non-fluoridated areas
[b]Mean age

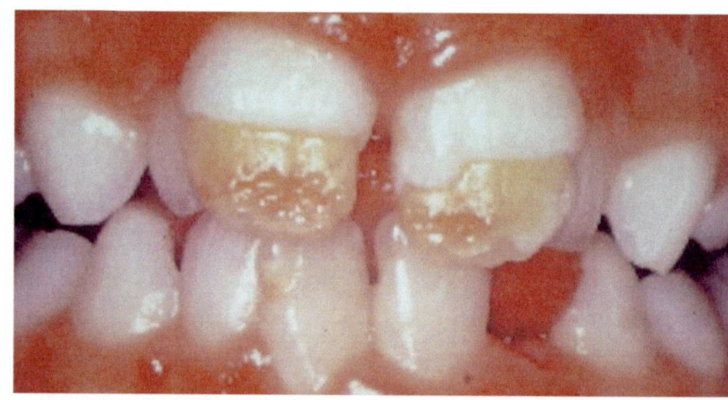

Fig. 2.1 Hypoplasia of the maxillary central incisors

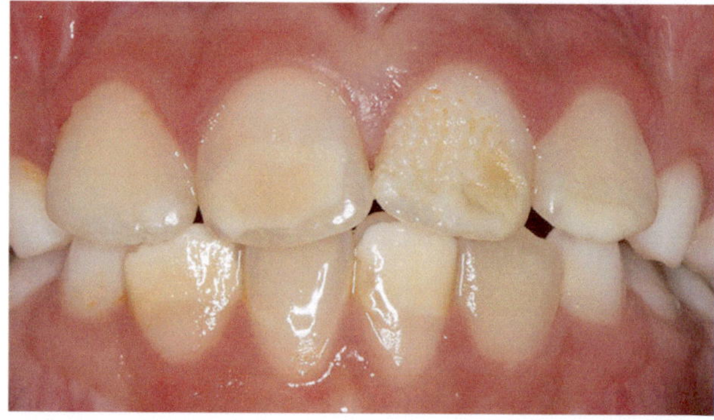

Fig. 2.2 Hypomineralization and hypoplasia of the maxillary and mandibular incisor teeth

of the incisors, progressing to the cervical areas of the teeth [29]. However, there is still limited understanding of how mineralization progresses across the crowns of the teeth. This could be important in determining the timing of defects to relate to specific disturbances caused by systemic disorders. Disturbances in the different stages of enamel formation may result in a range of enamel defects with quite different clinical appearances and structural changes. Defective formation of the enamel matrix results in hypoplasia, a *quantitative* defect, depicted by generalized thinning or pitting types of defects (Fig. 2.1). Defective calcification of an otherwise normal fully developed organic enamel matrix results in hypomineralization, a *qualitative* defect (Fig. 2.2). This is seen clinically as changes in color and

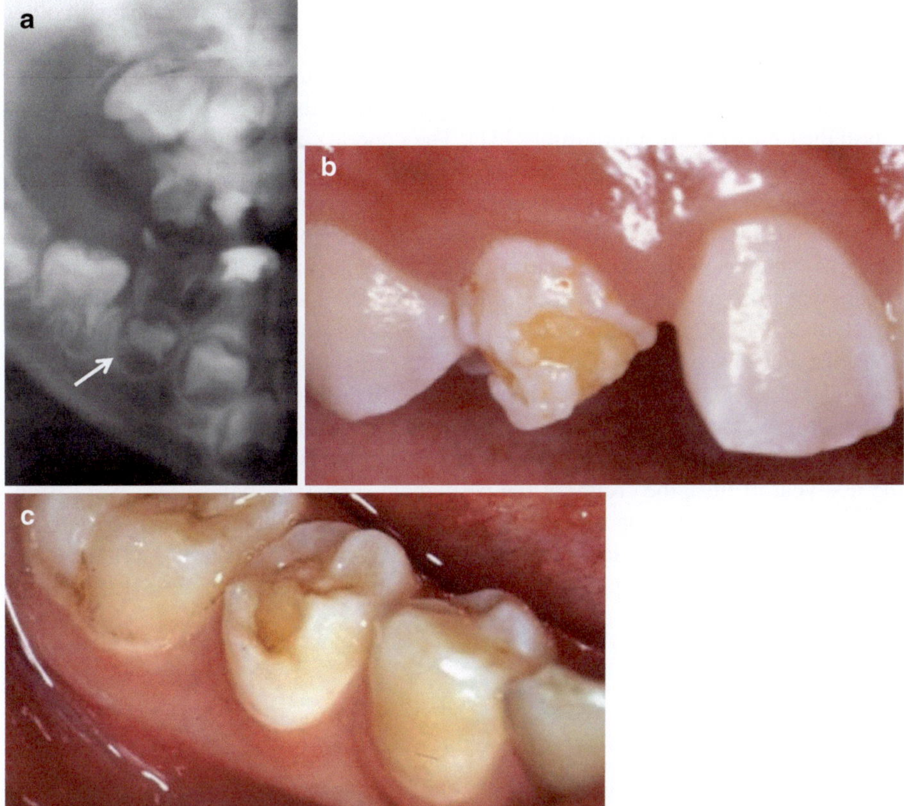

Fig. 2.3 (**a**) Caries in the mandibular second primary molar has led to the intra-radicular infection which has resulted in hypoplasia of the developing second premolar. (**b**) Hypoplasia of the maxillary permanent canine as a consequence of infection of the primary predecessor. (**c**) Hypoplasia in the form of missing enamel is exhibited by this mandibular second premolar following infection of the primary second molar

translucency of the enamel and presents as enamel opacities which can be either demarcated or diffuse [2, 30].

Although the etiology of enamel defects may be attributed to local, systemic, genetic, or environmental factors, most are likely to be multifactorial in nature. This makes it difficult to identify a single cause for many cases of DDE. The time frame of exposure and the mechanism underpinning the causative factors determine the presentation of these defects. Defects on a single tooth or only a few teeth suggest a local etiological factor e.g. a defect in a permanent tooth due to damage (trauma or infection) to its primary predecessor (Fig. 2.3a–c). Alternatively, a systemic factor (both short and longer term) may affect all the teeth that are developing during the time of the insult and lead to what is described as a chronological defect. Genetic factors can be considered separately. Defects caused by genetic factors are most often (although not always) generalized in distribution, affecting both the primary and permanent dentitions. They may present as either enamel defects alone as seen in amelogenesis imperfecta (see Chap. 5) or as enamel defects associated with other general genetic disorders/syndromes (see Chap. 4).

Enamel defects can be classified clinically as demarcated and diffuse opacities and hypoplasia. The location of isolated defects depends on the stage of amelogenesis at the time of the insult or injury [31]. The general consensus regarding the etiology of isolated opacities, which may be demarcated or diffuse and present as white, creamy, or yellow in color, is that amelogenesis is affected by a disturbance during the mineralization phase. It remains unclear why this would involve only an isolated patch of enamel on the crown and not the whole surface. Conversely, hypoplasia occurs when there is a disturbance during the secretory stage of amelogenesis while the enamel is only partly mineralized. Thus, enamel defects with similar presentations may have been caused by a variety of etiological factors. Furthermore, the same etiological factor can produce enamel defects with different presentations depending on the timing of the insult. Examples of this are commonly seen following primary tooth trauma. When a maxillary anterior primary tooth is intruded in infancy (during the first year of life), the crown of the permanent successor may suffer severe structural damage with missing enamel and even dilaceration of the root or the crown, while an intrusion in the later preschool years may only cause an isolated labial hypomineralized enamel opacity on the permanent successor (Fig. 2.4a, b).

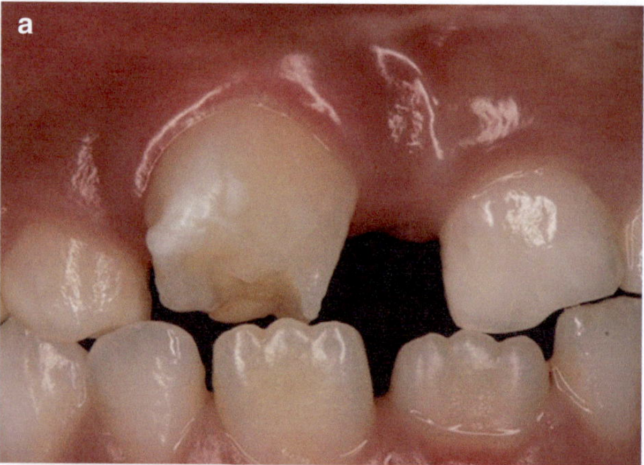

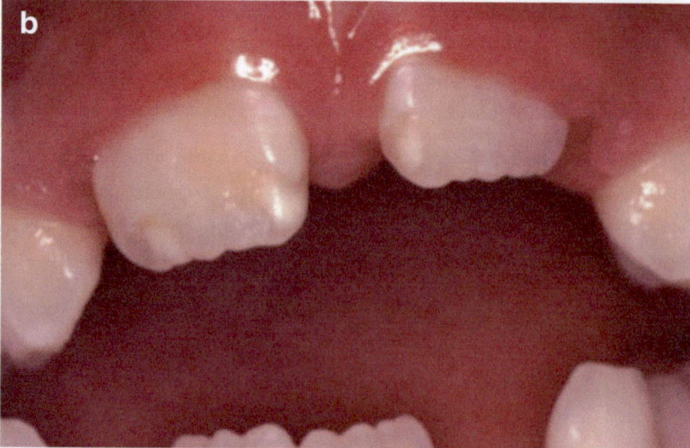

Fig. 2.4 (**a**) Hypoplasia of the maxillary permanent incisor tooth as a consequence of trauma to the predecessor. (**b**) Hypomineralization and hypoplasia of the maxillary central incisor teeth as a consequence of trauma to the predecessor

Determining the Etiology

Based on the number of teeth affected, the possible etiological factors for DDE in permanent teeth can be categorized as being local or general. However the evidence is equivocal, with the majority of published reports being animal studies or case reports of children with specific systemic disorders. The putative etiological factors reported in the literature are summarized in Table 2.3. Only a few of these factors have good evidence supporting a direct causal effect, e.g., trauma to a primary predecessor or high levels of ingested fluoride during early childhood.

Localized Enamel Defects

When only one or few adjacent teeth exhibit an enamel defect, it is usually considered to be caused by a very localized or isolated factor rather than a more generalized systemic or genetic factor [32]. The most common causes of localized enamel defects are trauma, chronic radicular infection resulting from pulpal necrosis in a primary predecessor tooth, surgery in the adjacent area or radiation therapy. Other isolated defects with incompletely formed enamel such as those associated with dens invaginatus and dens evaginatus may be due to a genetic influence in certain teeth.

Intrusive and lateral luxation injuries to the primary teeth often result in enamel defects in the succedaneous permanent teeth [33, 34]. This occurs most often in the anterior teeth as they are more likely to suffer the direct impact of trauma from falling or being struck by an object than the posterior teeth. The severe consequences arise because of the direct or nearly direct impact of the apex of the root of a primary incisor on the crown or follicle of the developing permanent successor or may occur as a consequence of post-traumatic complications of inflammation and infection. Furthermore, if the trauma to the primary tooth leads to pulpal necrosis, then there is a greater likelihood of enamel defects occurring in the succedaneous permanent tooth. This can also occur following severe dental caries with pulp exposure leading to untreated chronic infection [35]. Surgical procedures such as extraction of primary teeth, removal of supernumerary teeth, cleft palate repair or distraction osteogenesis have all been reported to cause localized enamel defects in the succedaneous or adjacent permanent teeth [36–39]. Untreated carious lesions extending into the pulp of primary teeth may result in pulpal necrosis and infection which may result in DDE in the succedaneous permanent teeth (Fig. 2.3) [40–42]. The reported defects have ranged from demarcated opacities to hypoplastic defects [43].

Generalized Enamel Defects

Generalized enamel defects are those defects that are seen either on the crowns of groups of teeth or in all the teeth. As mentioned previously, the stage of amelogenesis in the particular tooth germ at the time of the insult or injury is often critical to the resulting location and type of enamel defect. The timing of the disturbances

Table 2.3 List of etiological factors, reported in the literature, responsible for the formation of enamel defects in the permanent dentition

| Local | Systemic | | Hereditary conditions |
	Perinatal and neonatal	Postnatal	
Trauma Primary tooth Surgery Distraction osteogenesis Tooth forceps	Neonatal hypocalcemia	Nutritional and gastrointestinal disturbances resulting in hypocalcemia and vitamin D deficiency	22q11 deletion syndrome
Chronic periapical infection in a primary tooth	Severe perinatal and neonatal hypoxic injury	Bacterial and viral infections associated with high fever	Autoimmune polyendocrinopathy-candidiasis-ectodermal dystrophy
Cleft lip and palate	Prolonged delivery	Exanthematous diseases	Candidiasis endocrinopathy syndrome
Radiation	Prematurity	Juvenile hypothyroidism	Cleidocranial dysostosis
Burns	Low birth weight	Hypothyroidism	Celiac disease
Osteomyelitis	Twins	Hypogonadism	Congenital adrenal hyperplasia
Jaw fracture	Cerebral injury	Phenylketonuria	Congenital contractual arachnodactyly
	Neurological disorders	Alkaptonuria	Congenital unilateral facial hypoplasia
	Hyperbilirubinemia	Renal disorders	Ectodermal dysplasias
	Prolonged neonatal diarrhea and vomiting	Congenital heart disease	Ehlers-Danlos syndrome
	Severe neonatal infections	Congenital allergy	Epidermolysis bullosa
	High fever	Oxalosis	Focal dermal hypoplasia
		Mercury poisoning (acrodynia)	Heimler's syndrome
		Fluoride	Hypoparathyroidism
		Prolonged use of medicines	Ichthyosis vulgaris
		Prolonged diarrhea and vomiting	Lacrimo-auriculo-dento-digital syndrome
		Radiation and cytotoxic therapy	Morquio syndrome
			Mucopolysaccharidosis
			Oculodentodigital dysplasia
			Orodigitofacial dysostosis
			Prader-Willi syndrome
			Pseudohypoparathyroidism
			Seckel syndrome
			Tricho-dento-osseous syndrome
			Tuberous sclerosis
			Vitamin D-resistant rickets
			William's syndrome

during tooth morphogenesis will determine the location and type of defects and the number of teeth that will be affected. Homologous pairs of teeth will usually have enamel defects in similar locations although the severity of the defects may not always be the same suggesting that even homologous teeth do not always mineralize at exactly the same rate. As the process of enamel development occurs in the different tooth types over different developmental times, the locations of enamel defects will differ between different homologous pairs of teeth [44]. Developmental defects with this type of distribution are referred to as generalized defects of enamel and may be caused by environmental factors or systemic conditions that have either a defined time of influence or an ongoing influence throughout childhood, or they may be caused by genetic factors. These conditions and their association with DDE are discussed more fully in Chaps. 4 and 5.

Environmental Factors

Several environmental factors have been associated with DDE. These are believed to cause systemic disturbances that affect enamel development rather than the environmental agent affecting the ameloblasts directly. Environmental agents such as lead, mercury, bisphenol A (an endocrine-disrupting chemical), some drugs such as anticancer agents and tetracycline and some trace elements including fluoride and strontium have been implicated in DDE. The systemic ingestion of these chemical substances may exert an adverse effect on enamel formation during and after fetal development [45, 46]. Exposure to such substances during amelogenesis may result in the formation of defective enamel depending on the stage of enamel development, the timing of exposure, the length of exposure and the underlying health of the individual [47]. It should be remembered that some of the substances also have a very positive effect, such as the ingestion of low levels of fluoride to improve enamel maturation and decrease dental caries risk.

DDE arising from excess fluoride ingestion have been found in areas with high natural levels of fluoride in the drinking water. Ingestion of excess fluoride during tooth development can result in dental fluorosis, a form of enamel hypomineralization where the white striations contain less mineral and retain more developmental enamel proteins. The hypomineralization can vary from minor white striations to small or more extensive opacities [48, 49]. The first 3 years of life is generally understood to be the window of maximum susceptibility for the development of fluorosis in the permanent maxillary central incisor teeth [50]. Nevertheless, for the whole permanent dentition, excluding the third molars, the first 6–8 years of life is an important period when exposure to appropriate levels of fluoride as defined in local guidelines should be followed [51]. Fluorotic hypomineralization defects do have specific characteristics which allow them to be differentiated from defects caused by other factors [52], and this can be useful for the clinician to consider when diagnosing DDE. The characteristic lesions in fluorosis are dull and chalky in appearance; they may vary in color from chalky white, yellow, or brown, and in some cases there are small pits which accumulate organic matter producing yellow to brown spots (Fig. 2.5). When diagnosing DDE that

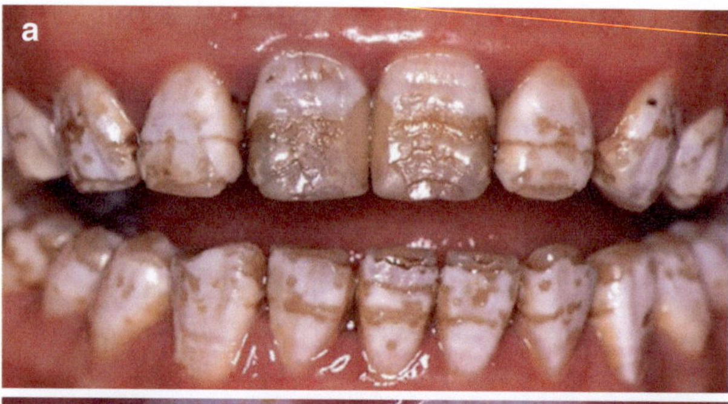
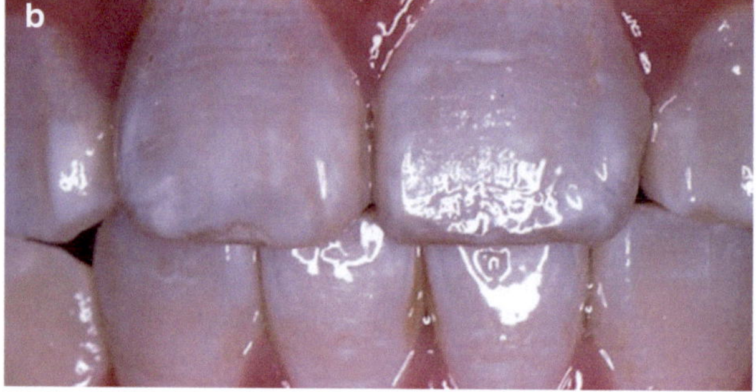

Fig. 2.5 (**a**) Fluorosis is evident in this permanent dentition of a child who was brought up in an area with 9 ppm of fluoride in the drinking water. (**b**) An example of less severe fluorosis

may be related to fluoride, a careful history of total fluoride ingestion as well as medical and developmental histories should be taken for the appropriate developmental period of the affected teeth. Another trace element that can have an influence on the development of hypomineralization in enamel is strontium which has been shown to be associated with enamel hypomineralization similar to that caused by excess fluoride [53].

Several animal experiments have shown that teeth are very sensitive to the effects of dioxins [54]. The most toxic dioxin, 2,3,7,8-tetrachlorodibenzo-para-dioxin (TCDD), arrests degradation and/or removal of enamel matrix proteins which is a pre-requisite for the completion of enamel mineralization [55]. It has been hypothesized that prolonged breast-feeding might increase the risk of DDE due to the environmental contamination of breast milk with dioxins or dioxin-like compounds [56, 57]. A dose-response relationship between high levels of dioxins or polychlorinated biphenyls (PCBs) exposure (serum concentration) and DDE in permanent teeth has been reported [58, 59]. However the evidence remains mixed with other studies reporting contradictory findings [11] and more recent studies failing to identify any correlation between DDE in children living in areas polluted by dioxins and in those living in areas with low pollution [60, 61]. It has also been reported that there is an increase in incidence of diffuse white/creamy mottling of enamel with elevated levels of chemicals such as fluorine, ammonia and sulfur in the atmosphere [62]; hypervitaminosis D [63]; chronic lead poisoning [64]; diphosphonate poisoning [65]; and polychlorinated biphenyl poisoning [66]. Antineoplastic therapy in the form of radiation treatment and/or chemotherapy can affect any cells including ameloblasts and consequently lead to DDE [67]. It has been reported that central nervous system irradiation with scattered irradiation of 0.72–1.44 Gy to the dental arches can result in a range of enamel defects in developing permanent teeth [68, 69].

Genetic Disorders

Amelogenesis imperfecta (AI) is a heterogeneous group of genetic disorders that affects the development of dental enamel resulting in varying degrees of hypoplasia, hypomineralization and/or hypomaturation [70]. A single-gene defect can occur as X-linked, autosomal dominant, or autosomal recessive inheritance. There is evidence that AI may present as part of a hereditary syndrome, examples of which are epidermolysis bullosa [71, 72], pseudohypoparathyroidism [73], and tricho-dento-osseous syndrome [74]. See Chaps. 4 and 5.

Systemic Conditions

It has been suggested that perinatal and postnatal problems, hypoxia and malnutrition may be related to the occurrence of DDE in permanent teeth. However, the mechanisms are not clearly understood and it is difficult to link any of the conditions directly to the defects. Children with low birth weights have been shown to be more at risk for developing DDE in their primary teeth. However the evidence is weaker in relation to the permanent dentition [75]. Similarly, problems at the time of delivery such as caesarean section and labor in excess of 20 h and poor respiratory response in the postnatal period (hypoxia and respiratory diseases in early childhood) have all been linked with the occurrence of DDE, but currently there is insufficient evidence to be confident about any of these as direct causes of DDE [76].

There are numerous reports of DDE in the permanent dentition being associated with diseases and infectious conditions occurring in early childhood. Infectious diseases occurring during early childhood that may be related to DDE include chickenpox, asthma, measles, mumps, scarlet fever, exanthematous fevers, pneumonia and urinary tract infections. Other conditions such as convulsions, tuberculosis, diphtheria, whooping cough, otitis media, bulbar polio with encephalitis, gastrointestinal disturbances, cyanotic congenital heart disease, neurological disorders and renal disorders have also all been mentioned in association with DDE.

Vitamin D deficiency, hypocalcemia, hypophosphatemia and hyperparathyroidism have also all be implicated in DDE in the permanent dentition. Vitamin D-dependent rickets (VDDR) is a condition which appears to be increasing in prevalence either due to vitamin D deficiency in the mother during pregnancy or vitamin D deficiency in the young child [77]. Vitamin D deficiency contributes to the development of hypocalcemia and hypophosphatemia which is then compounded by secondary hyperparathyroidism which in turn increases renal inorganic phosphate (P_i) clearance, effectively worsening the hypophosphatemia. Consequently the low concentrations of Ca^{2+} and P_i prevent proper mineralization of the organic bone matrix and this also leads to defects in enamel mineralization [78].

There is a growing body of literature reporting associations between DDE and systemic conditions such as celiac disease, cystic fibrosis and tuberous sclerosis though the mechanisms involved are often not fully understood [79–82]. Hypocalcemia has also associated with the occurrence of enamel hypoplasia in the permanent dentition in hereditary vitamin D-resistant rickets, X-linked hypophosphatemia, and hypoparathyroidism [83].

Despite the numerous reports of DDE in association with all of these conditions, there is little strong evidence to support any condition as being a primary etiological agent responsible for the formation of the enamel defects in the permanent dentition.

Summary

The prevalence of DDE in the permanent dentition (in developed countries) is reported to be between 9 and 68 %. This wide variation can be attributed to the use of different criteria and terminologies to describe enamel defects. The etiology of enamel defects may be local or systemic, genetic, or acquired in origin. The clinical presentation of DDE varies greatly depending on the etiology and severity. Single-tooth defects can be attributed to a local factor, whereas in those of systemic etiology many or all of the teeth that are developing during the time of influence of the etiological factor are affected (chronological defects). Defects with a genetic etiology form a separate entity, usually affecting both the primary and permanent teeth. Identifying the presence of DDE and establishing a diagnosis are essential to inform appropriate treatment planning in both the short and longer term (see Chap. 8).

References

1. AlQahtani SJ, Hector MP, Liversidge HM. Brief communication: the London atlas of human tooth development and eruption. Am J Phys Anthropol. 2010;142(3):481–90.
2. King N, Wei S. A review of the prevalence of developmental enamel defects in permanent teeth. J Paleopathol. 1992;2:342–57.
3. Suckling GW, Brown RH, Herbison GP. The prevalence of developmental defects of enamel in 696 nine-year-old New Zealand children participating in a health and development study. Community Dent Health. 1985;2(4):303–13.
4. Dooland MB, Wylie A. A photographic study of enamel defects among South Australian school children. Aust Dent J. 1989;34(5):470–3.
5. Dummer PM, Kingdon A, Kingdon R. Prevalence and distribution by tooth type and surface of developmental defects of dental enamel in a group of 15- to 16-year-old children in South Wales. Community Dent Health. 1990;7(4):369–77.
6. Nunn JH, Murray JJ, Reynolds P, Tabari D, Breckon J. The prevalence of developmental defects of enamel in 15–16-year-old children residing in three districts (natural fluoride, adjusted fluoride, low fluoride) in the north east of England. Community Dent Health. 1992;9(3):235–47.

7. Fyffe HE, Deery C, Pitts NB. Developmental defects of enamel in regularly attending adolescent dental patients in Scotland; prevalence and patient awareness. Community Dent Health. 1996;13(2):76–80.

8. Rugg-Gunn AJ, al-Mohammadi SM, Butler TJ. Effects of fluoride level in drinking water, nutritional status, and socio-economic status on the prevalence of developmental defects of dental enamel in permanent teeth in Saudi 14-year-old boys. Caries Res. 1997;31(4):259–67.

9. Hiller KA, Wilfart G, Schmalz G. Developmental enamel defects in children with different fluoride supplementation–a follow-up study. Caries Res. 1998;32(6):405–11.

10. Dini EL, Holt RD, Bedi R. Prevalence of caries and developmental defects of enamel in 9–10 year old children living in areas in Brazil with differing water fluoride histories. Br Dent J. 2000;188(3):146–9.

11. Jalevik B, Noren JG, Klingberg G, Barregard L. Etiologic factors influencing the prevalence of demarcated opacities in permanent first molars in a group of Swedish children. Eur J Oral Sci. 2001;109(4):230–4.

12. Zagdwon AM, Toumba KJ, Curzon ME. The prevalence of developmental enamel defects in permanent molars in a group of English school children. Eur J Paediatr Dent. 2002;3(2):91–6.

13. Ekanayake L, van der Hoek W. Prevalence and distribution of enamel defects and dental caries in a region with different concentrations of fluoride in drinking water in Sri Lanka. Int Dent J. 2003;53(4):243–8.

14. Cochran JA, Ketley CE, Arnadottir IB, Fernandes B, Koletsi-Kounari H, Oila AM, et al. A comparison of the prevalence of fluorosis in 8-year-old children from seven European study sites using a standardized methodology. Community Dent Oral Epidemiol. 2004;32 Suppl 1:28–33.

15. Mackay TD, Thomson WM. Enamel defects and dental caries among Southland children. N Z Dent J. 2005;101(2):35–43.

16. Balmer RC, Laskey D, Mahoney E, Toumba KJ. Prevalence of enamel defects and MIH in non-fluoridated and fluoridated communities. Eur J Paediatr Dent. 2005;6(4):209–12.

17. Wong HM, McGrath C, Lo EC, King NM. Association between developmental defects of enamel and different concentrations of fluoride in the public water supply. Caries Res. 2006;40(6):481–6.

18. Hoffmann RH, de Sousa Mda L, Cypriano S. Prevalence of enamel defects and the relationship to dental caries in deciduous and permanent dentition in Indaiatuba, Sao Paulo, Brazil. Cad Saude Publica. 2007;23(2):435–44.

19. Muratbegovic A, Zukanovic A, Markovic N. Molar-incisor-hypomineralisation impact on developmental defects of enamel prevalence in a low fluoridated area. Eur Arch Paediatr Dent. 2008;9(4):228–31.

20. Arrow P. Prevalence of developmental enamel defects of the first permanent molars among school children in Western Australia. Aust Dent J. 2008;53(3):250–9.

21. Kanagaratnam S, Schluter P, Durward C, Mahood R, Mackay T. Enamel defects and dental caries in 9-year-old children living in fluoridated and nonfluoridated areas of Auckland, New Zealand. Community Dent Oral Epidemiol. 2009;37(3):250–9.

22. Seow WK, Ford D, Kazoullis S, Newman B, Holcombe T. Comparison of enamel defects in the primary and permanent dentitions of children from a low-fluoride District in Australia. Pediatr Dent. 2011;33(3):207–12.

23. Casanova-Rosado AJ, Medina-Solis CE, Casanova-Rosado JF, Vallejos-Sanchez AA, Martinez-Mier EA, Loyola-Rodriguez JP, et al. Association between developmental enamel defects in the primary and permanent dentitions. Eur J Paediatr Dent. 2011;12(3):155–8.

24. Robles MJ, Ruiz M, Bravo-Perez M, Gonzalez E, Penalver MA. Prevalence of enamel defects in primary and permanent teeth in a group of schoolchildren from Granada (Spain). Med Oral Patol Oral Cir Bucal. 2013;18(2):e187–93.

25. Vargas-Ferreira F, Zeng J, Thomson WM, Peres MA, Demarco FF. Association between developmental defects of enamel and dental caries in schoolchildren. J Dent. 2014;42(5):540–6.

26. Angelillo IF, Romano F, Fortunato L, Montanaro D. Prevalence of dental caries and enamel defects in children living in areas with different water fluoride concentrations. Community Dent Health. 1990;7(3):229–36.
27. Suckling GW, Pearce EI. Developmental defects of enamel in a group of New Zealand children: their prevalence and some associated etiological factors. Community Dent Oral Epidemiol. 1984;12(3):177–84.
28. de Liefde B, Herbison GP. Prevalence of developmental defects of enamel and dental caries in New Zealand children receiving differing fluoride supplementation. Community Dent Oral Epidemiol. 1985;13(3):164–7.
29. Hillson S, Bond S. Relationship of enamel hypoplasia to the pattern of tooth crown growth: a discussion. Am J Phys Anthropol. 1997;104(1):89–103.
30. King N. Prevalence and characteristics of developmental defects of dental enamel in Hong Kong. PhD thesis, The University of Hong Kong; 1990.
31. Giro CM. Enamel hypoplasia in human teeth; an examination of its causes. J Am Dent Assoc. 1947;34(5):310–7.
32. Jorgenson RJ, Yost C. Etiology of enamel dysplasia. J Pedod. 1982;6(4):315–29.
33. Sleiter R, von Arx T. Developmental disorders of permanent teeth after injuries of their primary predecessors. A retrospective study. Schweiz Monatsschr Zahnmed. 2002;112(3):214–9.
34. Hall S, Iranpour B. The effect of trauma on normal tooth development. Report of two cases. ASDC J Dent Child. 1968;35(4):291–5.
35. Holan G, Topf J, Fuks AB. Effect of root canal infection and treatment of traumatized primary incisors on their permanent successors. Endod Dent Traumatol. 1992;8(1):12–5.
36. Dixon DA. Defects of structure and formation of the teeth in persons with cleft palate and the effect of reparative surgery on the dental tissues. Oral Surg Oral Med Oral Pathol. 1968;25(3):435–46.
37. Kleine-Hakala M, Hukki J, Hurmerinta K. Effect of mandibular distraction osteogenesis on developing molars. Orthod Craniofac Res. 2007;10(4):196–202.
38. Ranta R. A review of tooth formation in children with cleft lip/palate. Am J Orthod Dentofacial Orthop. 1986;90(1):11–8.
39. Williamson JJ. Trauma during exodontia. An aetiologic factor in hypoplastic premolars. Br Dent J. 1966;121(6):284–9.
40. Kimoto S, Suga H, Yamaguchi M, Uchimura N, Ikeda M, Kakizawa T. Hypoplasia of primary and permanent teeth following osteitis and the implications of delayed diagnosis of a neonatal maxillary primary molar. Int J Paediatr Dent. 2003;13(1):35–40.
41. McCormick J, Filostrat DJ. Injury to the teeth of succession by abscess of the temporary teeth. J Dent Child. 1967;34(6):501–4.
42. Turner J. Effects of abscess arising from temporary teeth. Br J Dent Sci. 1906;49:562–4.
43. Brook AH, Winter GB. Developmental arrest of permanent tooth germs following pulpal infection of deciduous teeth. Br Dent J. 1975;139(1):9–11.
44. Lunt RC, Law DB. A review of the chronology of calcification of deciduous teeth. J Am Dent Assoc. 1974;89(3):599–606.
45. Knothe H, Dette GA. Antibiotics in pregnancy: toxicity and teratogenicity. Infection. 1985;13(2):49–51.
46. Phillips-Howard PA, Wood D. The safety of antimalarial drugs in pregnancy. Drug Saf. 1996;14(3):131–45.
47. Billings RJ, Berkowitz RJ, Watson G. Teeth. Pediatrics. 2004;113(4 Suppl):1120–7.
48. Fejerskov O, Larsen MJ, Richards A, Baelum V. Dental tissue effects of fluoride. Adv Dent Res. 1994;8(1):15–31.
49. Rozier RG. Epidemiologic indices for measuring the clinical manifestations of dental fluorosis: overview and critique. Adv Dent Res. 1994;8(1):39–55.
50. Hong L, Levy SM, Warren JJ, Broffitt B, Cavanaugh J. Fluoride intake levels in relation to fluorosis development in permanent maxillary central incisors and first molars. Caries Res. 2006;40(6):494–500.

51. Pendrys DG, Stamm JW. Relationship of total fluoride intake to beneficial effects and enamel fluorosis. J Dent Res. 1990;69 Spec No:529–38. Discussion 56–7.
52. Cutress TW, Suckling GW. Differential diagnosis of dental fluorosis. J Dent Res. 1990;69 Spec No:714–20. Discussion 21.
53. Curzon ME, Spector PC. Enamel mottling in a high strontium area of the U.S.A. Community Dent Oral Epidemiol. 1977;5(5):243–7.
54. Alaluusua S, Lukinmaa PL. Developmental dental toxicity of dioxin and related compounds–a review. Int Dent J. 2006;56(6):323–31.
55. Gao Y, Sahlberg C, Kiukkonen A, Alaluusua S, Pohjanvirta R, Tuomisto J, et al. Lactational exposure of Han/Wistar rats to 2,3,7,8-tetrachlorodibenzo-p-dioxin interferes with enamel maturation and retards dentin mineralization. J Dent Res. 2004;83(2):139–44.
56. Alaluusua S, Lukinmaa PL, Koskimies M, Pirinen S, Holtta P, Kallio M, et al. Developmental dental defects associated with long breast feeding. Eur J Oral Sci. 1996;104(5–6):493–7.
57. Alaluusua S, Lukinmaa PL, Vartiainen T, Partanen M, Torppa J, Tuomisto J. Polychlorinated dibenzo-p-dioxins and dibenzofurans via mother's milk may cause developmental defects in the child's teeth. Environ Toxicol Pharmacol. 1996;1(3):193–7.
58. Alaluusua S, Calderara P, Gerthoux PM, Lukinmaa PL, Kovero O, Needham L, et al. Developmental dental aberrations after the dioxin accident in Seveso. Environ Health Perspect. 2004;112(13):1313–8.
59. Jan J, Sovcikova E, Kocan A, Wsolova L, Trnovec T. Developmental dental defects in children exposed to PCBs in eastern Slovakia. Chemosphere. 2007;67(9):S350–4.
60. Kuscu OO, Caglar E, Aslan S, Durmusoglu E, Karademir A, Sandalli N. The prevalence of molar incisor hypomineralization (MIH) in a group of children in a highly polluted urban region and a windfarm-green energy island. Int J Paediatr Dent. 2009;19(3):176–85.
61. Laisi S, Kiviranta H, Lukinmaa PL, Vartiainen T, Alaluusua S. Molar-incisor-hypomineralisation and dioxins: new findings. Eur Arch Paediatr Dent. 2008;9(4):224–7.
62. Wozniak K. Developmental abnormalities of mineralization in populations with varying exposure to fluorine compounds. Ann Acad Med Stetin. 2000;46:305–15.
63. Giunta JL. Dental changes in hypervitaminosis D. Oral Surg Oral Med Oral Pathol Oral Radiol Endod. 1998;85(4):410–3.
64. Lawson BF, Stout FW, Ahern DE, Sneed WD. The incidence of enamel hypoplasia associated with chronic pediatric lead poisoning. S C Dent J. 1971;29(11):5–10.
65. Fouda N, Caracatsanis M, Hammarstrom L. Developmental disturbances of the rat molar induced by two diphosphonates. Adv Dent Res. 1989;3(2):234–40.
66. Jan J, Vrbic V. Polychlorinated biphenyls cause developmental enamel defects in children. Caries Res. 2000;34(6):469–73.
67. Minicucci EM, Lopes LF, Crocci AJ. Dental abnormalities in children after chemotherapy treatment for acute lymphoid leukemia. Leuk Res. 2003;27(1):45–50.
68. Duggal MS, Curzon ME, Bailey CC, Lewis IJ, Prendergast M. Dental parameters in the long-term survivors of childhood cancer compared with siblings. Oral Oncol. 1997;33(5):348–53.
69. Pajari U, Lanning M. Developmental defects of teeth in survivors of childhood ALL are related to the therapy and age at diagnosis. Med Pediatr Oncol. 1995;24(5):310–4.
70. Crawford PJ, Aldred M, Bloch-Zupan A. Amelogenesis imperfecta. Orphanet J Rare Dis. 2007;2:17.
71. Arwill T, Olsson O, Bergenholtz A. Epidermolysis bullosa hereditaria. 3. A histologic study of changes in teeth in the polydysplastic dystrophic and lethal forms. Oral Surg Oral Med Oral Pathol. 1965;19:723–44.
72. Wright JT, Johnson LB, Fine JD. Development defects of enamel in humans with hereditary epidermolysis bullosa. Arch Oral Biol. 1993;38(11):945–55.
73. Jensen SB, Illum F, Dupont E. Nature and frequency of dental changes in idiopathic hypoparathyroidism and pseudohypoparathyroidism. Scand J Dent Res. 1981;89(1):26–37.
74. Spangler GS, Hall KI, Kula K, Hart TC, Wright JT. Enamel structure and composition in the tricho-dento-osseous syndrome. Connect Tissue Res. 1998;39(1–3):165–75. Discussion 87–94.

75. Jacobsen PE, Haubek D, Henriksen TB, Ostergaard JR, Poulsen S. Developmental enamel defects in children born preterm: a systematic review. Eur J Oral Sci. 2014;122(1):7–14.
76. Beentjes VE, Weerheijm KL, Groen HJ. Factors involved in the aetiology of molar-incisor hypomineralisation (MIH). Eur J Paediatr Dent. 2002;3(1):9–13.
77. Bell DS. Protean manifestations of vitamin D deficiency, part 1: the epidemic of deficiency. South Med J. 2011;104(5):331–4.
78. Foster BL, Nociti Jr FH, Somerman MJ. The rachitic tooth. Endocr Rev. 2014;35(1):1–34.
79. Flanagan N, O'Connor WJ, McCartan B, Miller S, McMenamin J, Watson R. Developmental enamel defects in tuberous sclerosis: a clinical genetic marker? J Med Genet. 1997;34(8):637–9.
80. Narang A, Maguire A, Nunn JH, Bush A. Oral health and related factors in cystic fibrosis and other chronic respiratory disorders. Arch Dis Child. 2003;88(8):702–7.
81. Rasmusson CG, Eriksson MA. Celiac disease and mineralisation disturbances of permanent teeth. Int J Paediatr Dent. 2001;11(3):179–83.
82. Wierink CD, van Diermen DE, Aartman IH, Heymans HS. Dental enamel defects in children with coeliac disease. Int J Paediatr Dent. 2007;17(3):163–8.
83. Zambrano M, Nikitakis NG, Sanchez-Quevedo MC, Sauk JJ, Sedano H, Rivera H. Oral and dental manifestations of vitamin D-dependent rickets type I: report of a pediatric case. Oral Surg Oral Med Oral Pathol Oral Radiol Endod. 2003;95(6):705–9.

Molar Incisor Hypomineralization and Hypomineralized Second Primary Molars: Diagnosis, Prevalence, and Etiology

3

Karin L. Weerheijm, Marlies E.C. Elfrink,
and Nicky Kilpatrick

Abstract

Molar incisor hypomineralization (MIH) is a term used to describe a specific clinical entity in which there are demarcated opacities in erupting first permanent molars, frequently in combination with similar opacities in permanent incisors. Recently, comparable lesions have been reported in second primary molars and are referred to as hypomineralized second primary molars (HSPM). This chapter describes the diagnosis, etiology, and prevalence of MIH and HSPM and discusses the clinical characteristics and implications of this subgroup of DDE. Given the specific distribution of the developmental defects associated with MIH (and HSPM), the timing of any causative environmental disruption can be hypothesized to be between the 18th week of pregnancy and around 3–5 years of age. However, the evidence surrounding specific factors remains weak, not least because of a lack of consensus regarding assessment protocols and limited understanding as to the exact pathogenesis. Etiology seems to be multifactorial, and the etiological factors can be found in the pre-, peri-, and postnatal period. The literature suggests the worldwide prevalence of MIH varies

K.L. Weerheijm, PhD (✉)
Department of Cariology Endodontology Pedodontology, Academic Centre for Dentistry (ACTA),
Paediatric Dentist, Kindertand Zuid and Member Paediatric Research Project (PREP),
Milletstraat 28 hs, Amsterdam 1077 ZE, The Netherlands
e-mail: weerkamp@xs4all.nl

M.E.C. Elfrink, PhD
Department of Cariology Endodontology Pedodontology, Academic Centre for Dentistry (ACTA),
Paediatric Dentist, Mondzorgcentrum Nijverdal and Member Paediatric
Research Project (PREP), Stationsstraat 7, Nijverdal 7443 BX, The Netherlands
e-mail: marlieselfrink@gmail.com

N. Kilpatrick, BDS, PhD
Cleft and Craniofacial Research, Murdoch Childrens Research Institute,
Flemington Road, Parkville, Melbourne, VIC 3052, Australia
e-mail: nicky@bassdata.com.au

© Springer-Verlag Berlin Heidelberg 2015
B.K. Drummond, N. Kilpatrick (eds.), *Planning and Care for Children and Adolescents with Dental Enamel Defects: Etiology, Research and Contemporary Management*, DOI 10.1007/978-3-662-44800-7_3

between 2.8 % and 44 %, whereas for HSPM, figures of between 4.9 and 9.0 % have been reported. The presence of HSPM and demarcated opacities in erupting permanent incisors represents risk indicators for subsequent MIH. As MIH is associated with hypersensitive teeth, posteruptive loss of enamel and rapid caries progression early diagnosis is clinically very important.

Introduction

Despite a general decline in caries prevalence over the past 30 years, there remains a subgroup of children in whom rapid caries progression, particularly affecting the first permanent and second deciduous molars, still occurs. These children present frequently to dentists who are confronted with large defects during or soon after the eruption of the affected teeth. In 1987 Koch et al. [1] reported the prevalence of hypomineralized first permanent molars in different Swedish birth cohorts. These molars have subsequently been referred to in the literature, as non-fluoride hypomineralization, idiopathic enamel hypomineralization, non-endemic mottling of enamel, or cheese molars [2]. The phenomenon, known as molar incisor hypomineralization (MIH) was first recognized in 2001 and defined as hypomineralization of one to four first permanent molars often in combination with affected permanent incisors (Fig. 3.1) [3]. Subsequently, MIH-like lesions have been recognized in second primary molars (Fig. 3.2) leading to the description of hypomineralized second primary molars (HSPM) [4] also called deciduous molar hypomineralization (DMH) [5].

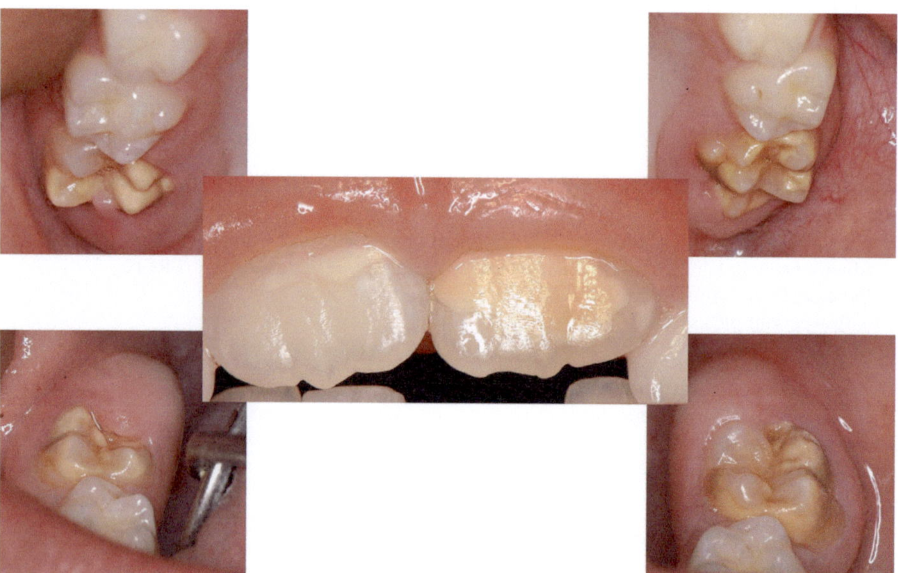

Fig. 3.1 Example of MIH with molar as well as incisor opacities. Notice the *white* demarcated opacity 11, *yellow* demarcated opacity 21. *Yellow brown* demarcated opacities erupting 46, *brown* demarcated opacities with occlusal buccal posteruptive enamel loss 36, as well as demarcated *yellow brown* opacities in erupting 16 and 26 (Courtesy of Dr. H. Pohlen, Alsdorf, Germany)

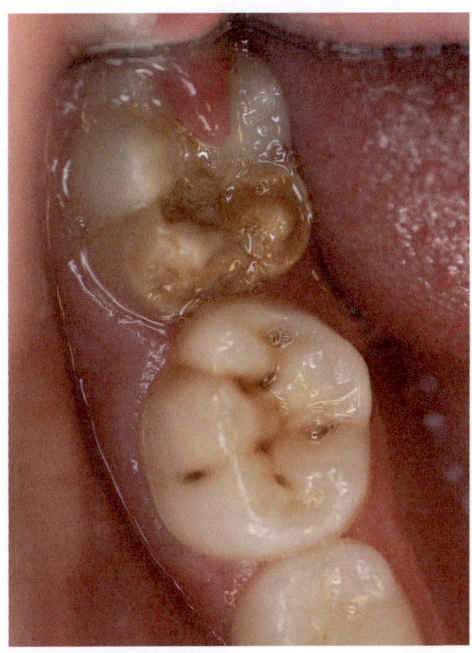

Fig. 3.2 Mild HSPM in the 85 while the erupting 46 shows already severe MIH (posteruptive enamel loss on both mesial cusps)

Diagnostic Criteria

In 2003, following a consensus meeting of the European Academy of Pediatric Dentistry (EAPD), criteria for epidemiological studies of MIH were developed including recognition of the potential for MIH-like hypomineralization defects to occur in second primary molars [4]. In 2009 in Helsinki, the EAPD updated these criteria [6] such that currently the criteria for MIH include demarcated opacities, posteruptive breakdown (or PEB) and both atypical restorations and extractions of the permanent molars and/or incisors. HSPM is defined similarly as hypomineralization of one to four second primary molars [7, 8]. To diagnose HSPM, the same criteria are used as for MIH with "atypical caries" being included in addition to "atypical restorations." Especially in the primary dentition, cavities may not be restored in certain populations.

To arrive at a diagnosis of MIH, it is important to identify white, yellow or brown demarcated opacities on at least one first permanent molar. The greater the number of affected molars in an individual patient the greater the risk that the incisors will also be affected [2, 9]. The presence of opacities on the permanent incisors is *not* mandatory for the diagnosis of MIH. However, opacities that *only* occur on permanent incisors do not lead to a diagnosis of MIH. This is because the etiology of opacities confined to permanent incisors is likely to be different to that of the more widespread MIH condition. Traumatic injuries (particularly intrusive ones) to primary incisors impact on the developing tooth germs and commonly lead to localized anomalies of the permanent successors [2, 4, 10].

Clinical Features

MIH is a hypomineralization defect affecting the quality (as opposed to the quantity) of the enamel. It is identified visually as an alteration in translucency of the enamel, with a sharp demarcation between the affected and sound enamel, known as a demarcated opacity. The color of the hypomineralized area is white, yellow or brown and the area has a dull (porous) or shiny surface appearance (Fig. 3.3). MIH is not only variable in expression between patients but also within an individual patient. The number of affected first permanent molars per child can vary from one to four and the expression of the defects may vary from molar to molar. Within one patient, intact demarcated opacities can be found in one molar, while in another molar in the same patient, the porous enamel is already broken down (asymmetrical appearance). The porous brittle enamel can easily chip off under the masticatory forces very soon after eruption. This chipping off has been described in the literature as posteruptive enamel loss or PEB [4]. Sometimes the loss of enamel in PEB can occur so rapidly after eruption that it seems as if it was not formed initially (Fig. 3.4). However, it is important that the clinician distinguishes between PEB and hypoplasia. Hypoplasia is a primary quantitative defect of the enamel that occurs during tooth development. The resulting enamel may be thin or actually missing and may be characterized as pits or grooves across the tooth surface. The color and location of the demarcated opacities in MIH-affected molars are indicative of the

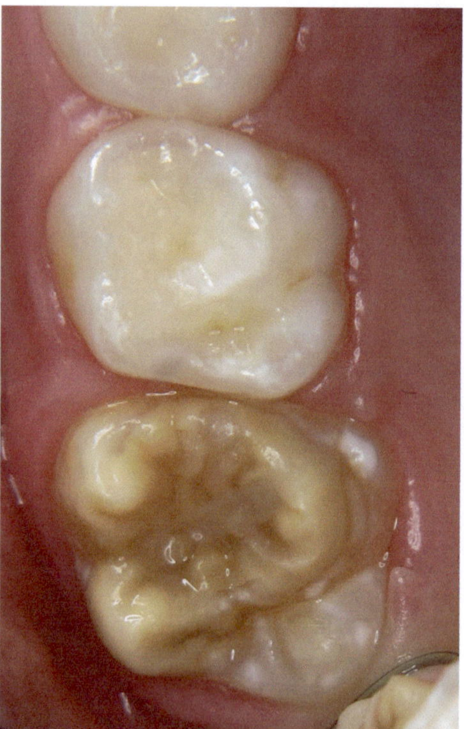

Fig. 3.3 *Yellow* to *brown* demarcated opacity covering almost the entire occlusal surface of the recently erupted 16 (Courtesy of Dr. M. van Ulsen, Amsterdam, the Netherlands)

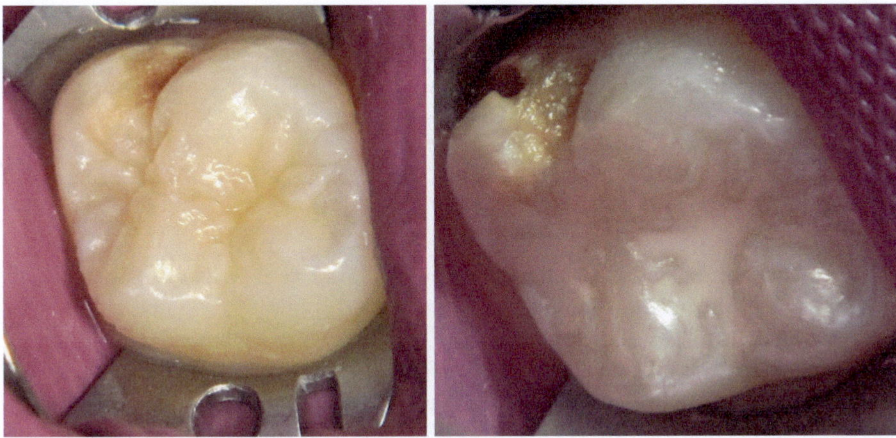

Fig. 3.4 Tooth 16 with posteruptive enamel loss and opacity on the palatal surface. The same tooth after 1 year posteruptive enamel loss with cavity formation

Fig. 3.5 Incisors with demarcated opacities in a child with severe MIH. Notice the *white* opacities in teeth 31 and 41, the *light yellow/white* opacities in teeth 11 and 21, and the *dark yellow* opacities in the 32 and 42

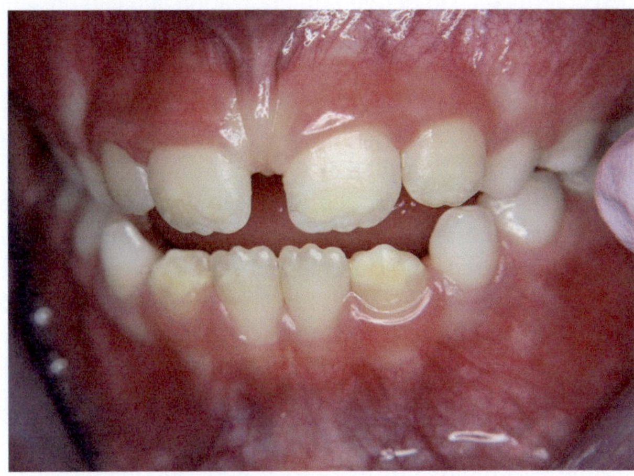

relative risk for PEB; brown, dull, and porous opacities on cuspal tips are thought to be weaker than white and shiny ones on smooth surfaces and therefore more vulnerable to chipping [9].

The clinical appearance of the location, size, and form of the HSPM- and MIH-related carious lesions and restorations often do not fit with normal caries distribution patterns. These lesions and restorations have been reported as atypical caries or atypical restorations in some epidemiological studies [4]. When the incisors also show opacities most commonly these remain intact because the chewing forces have less impact on incisors compared with molars (Fig. 3.5).

Both MIH and HSPM are very inconvenient for the child. The child may experience pain and sensitivity from the affected teeth particularly when exposed to hot and cold foods and drinks. Even if the (porous) hypomineralized enamel is intact, toothbrushing can cause sensitivity [2, 3]. In the event of PEB caries can progress rapidly increasing the risk of toothache. Pain-free treatment, which can be challenging because the teeth are sensitive, is important to avoid behavioral management problems or the development of dental anxiety in the future [11].

Etiology of MIH

Tooth development is under strict genetic control; however it is also very sensitive to environmental changes. Ameloblasts, which are highly specialized calcium-transporting cells, play an integral role in all three of the stages of enamel formation: matrix formation, initial calcification and final maturation [12]. If ameloblast function is disrupted during the secretory phase, there will be irreversible damage to the cells and the teeth are characterized by a deficiency of tooth substance that ranges from minor pits and groves to total absence of enamel; this is termed enamel hypoplasia and is a quantitative defect. If, however, disruption of ameloblasts occurs later during either the calcification or maturation phase, then the teeth will manifest in a qualitative defect termed enamel hypomineralization and can present as an enamel opacity [13].

As discussed in Chaps. 1 and 2, ameloblasts are highly susceptible to environmental disruptions leading to developmental defects in the enamel (DDE). Depending on the timing of the disruption, which can be from the time the first primary tooth starts to form (15–19 weeks in utero) to the completion of the maturation of the third permanent molar (around 12 years of age), the defects manifest differently across either dentition. However MIH is a very distinct form of DDE in which the enamel of the first permanent molars (+/− the incisors) is specifically hypomineralized. First permanent molars begin to develop in the fourth month in utero, but calcification does not start until around the time of birth. For an environmental disruption to contribute to MIH specifically, it would therefore likely occur from sometime around the time of birth to 3–5 years of age by which time maturation of the coronal enamel on the first permanent molars (and incisors) is complete. Recent in vitro studies have suggested an even narrower window of susceptibility around 6–8 months of age based upon the histological, mechanical, and chemical properties of affected first molar teeth [14, 15]. In general, the putative causes of MIH are similar to those identified in Chaps. 1 and 2 in association with more generalized DDE in both the primary and permanent dentitions. Table 3.1 is a summary of the possible etiological factors for MIH. The factors are divided into pre-, peri- and postnatal factors with medical problems being commonly mentioned. Fluoride does not appear to influence the occurrence of MIH [25].

The strength of the evidence surrounding the etiology of MIH specifically remains weak [18, 25]. There are a number of reasons for this including:

(i) The historical lack of consensus surrounding both the definition of MIH and how to record it, leading to the use of a wide variety of often unvalidated indices.
(ii) Reliance on retrospective data either using parental recall of the perinatal period or, slightly more reliable but nevertheless generally incomplete, retrospective chart reviews.

Table 3.1 Factors *putatively* associated with MIH

			Factor	Reference
Prenatal				
Lifestyle	Health		Maternal illness or infection	[16, 17]
			Maternal hypocalcemia	[16, 17]
			Nutrition	[16, 18, 19]
Perinatal				
	Health		Infant hypoxia	[16, 18, 20, 21]
			Very low birth weight	[22, 23]
			Premature birth	[18, 21, 24]
			Calcium shortage	[16, 18, 19]
			Misc medical problems	[18]
Postnatal				
	Lifestyle		Breastfeeding	[14, 17, 18, 21, 25–27]
			Nutrition	[14, 19]
			Calcium shortage	[16, 18, 19]
	Environment		Dioxins and polychlorinated bisphenols	[1, 18, 25, 26, 28–35]
			Environmental pollution	[31, 33]
	Health		Childhood illnesses (in general)	[16–18, 21, 25, 26, 36]
			Chicken pox and other viral infections	[17]
			Otitis media	[21, 26]
			Asthma, lung problems, allergy	[17, 21, 26, 37]
			Fevers (irrespective of cause)	[21, 38]
			Medications (in general)	[17, 18, 25, 26, 39]
			Antibiotics	[17, 39–41]
			Antiasthmatic medication	[42]

(iii) Under-recording of the problem. First permanent molars affected by MIH are susceptible to both PEB and rapid carious attack shortly after emerging into the oral cavity. Many studies exclude restored or carious teeth from the assessment which is likely to lead to an under-reporting of MIH, while others may incorrectly classify PEB as hypoplasia. Similarly, severely affected molars often require early extraction. Many studies include population samples of children over 10 years old and few make any attempt to discover why missing teeth have been extracted – this is also likely to lead to under-reporting of MIH.

A further confounding factor when attempting to unravel the etiology of MIH is how to account for the typically asymmetric distribution of the hypomineralized lesions in MIH. This makes it difficult to attribute definitive causality between an environmental disruption and the presence of MIH. This may be explained in part by variations in the timing of mineralization of homologous pairs of teeth i.e. lower second molars [43]. It is also possible that there are genetic factors [44, 45] and local environmental factors within developing tooth germs themselves that may predispose to MIH. As understanding of the structure and composition of MIH-affected enamel evolves the etiology of this condition will become clearer but is almost certainly multifactorial and complex.

Etiology of HSPM

As with MIH, the etiology of HSPM appears to be multifactorial. Three studies have been published to date with the pre- and perinatal factors being reportedly more important in HSPM than in MIH [46–48]. Ninety-four percent of children with HSPM have been reported to have at least one medical problem: 24.5 % occurring prenatally, 45.3 % perinatally, and 9.4 % postnatally [46] with the greater the number of medical problems the greater the risk of HSPM. Furthermore, the ethnicity of the child, maternal alcohol consumption during pregnancy, low birth weight and fever episodes in the child's first year of life have been identified as risk factors for HSPM [47]. Conversely, use of medications during pregnancy (specifically antibiotics and antiasthmatic and anti-allergic medications) does not seem to influence the occurrence of HSPM [47, 48].

Prevalence of MIH

The reported prevalence of MIH varies between 2.8 and 44 %. However despite the publication of recommended diagnostic criteria for [4, 6], the lack of consensus surrounding examination protocols, choice of index and population characteristics means that it is still hard to make valid comparisons between the various epidemiological studies [14, 25]. Table 3.2 summarizes the reported prevalence of MIH worldwide including the indices used in each study. In addition to differences in reported prevalence of MIH between countries, differences are also noted across birth year. For example, in the study of Koch et al. [1], the prevalence of MIH varied between 4.4 and 15.4 % across the different birth years with a peak in prevalence for those children born in 1970. These data were reproduced later by Jalevik et al. in Swedish children born in 1990 [26]. Most studies show an equal distribution of MIH between sexes [26, 55, 71] and, although Leppäniemi et al. [55] found a predisposition for MIH in the upper jaw, most studies fail to show any quadrant predilection for MIH defects [9, 26, 68, 71].

Prevalence of HSPM

Compared with MIH, there are very few prevalence studies on HSPM. Table 3.3 summarizes the available data which suggests that the prevalence of HSPM varies between 4.9 and 9.0 %. HSPM is also equally distributed between sexes and arches [7]. HSPM is now also recognized as a risk factor and clinical indicator for MIH (OR: 4.4 (95 % CI: 3.1–6.4) [72]. Even relatively mild expressions of HSPM increase the chances of future MIH (Fig. 3.2) [72]. In children with mild HSPM, the

Table 3.2 Overview of the prevalence studies on MIH

Country	Prevalence (%)	Score criteria	Reference
Australia	22	mDDE	Arrow [49]
Australia	44	mDDE	Balmer et al. [50]
Bosnia and Herzegovina	12.3	EAPD 2003	Muratbegovic et al. [51]
Brazil	40.2	EAPD 2003	Soviero et al. [52]
Brazil	19.8	EAPD 2003	da Costa-Silva et al. [53]
China/Hong Kong	2.8	EAPD 2003	Cho et al. [54]
Denmark	37.3	EAPD 2003	Wogelius et al. [42]
Finland	17	Alaluusua 1996	Alaluusua et al. [30]
Finland	19.3	Alaluusua 1996	Leppaniemi et al. [55]
Germany	9.9	EAPD 2003	Petrou et al. [56]
Greece	10.2	EAPD 2003	Lygidakis et al. [16]
India	9.2	EAPD 2003	Parikh et al. [57]
Iran	20.2	EAPD 2003	Ghanim et al. [58]
Iraq	21.5	EAPD 2003	Ghanim et al. [59]
Italy	13.7	MIH 2001	Calderara et al. [60]
Jordan	17.6	EAPD 2003	Zawaideh et al. [61]
Libia	2.9	MIH 2001	Fteita et al. [62]
Lithuania	9.7	EAPD 2003	Jasulaityte et al. [63]
New Zealand	14.9	mDDE	Mahoney and Morrison [64]
New Zealand	18.8	mDDE	Mahoney and Morrison [65]
Spain	17.8	EAPD 2003	Martínez Gómez et al. [66]
Spain	21.8	EAPD 2003	Garcia-Margarit et al. [67]
Sweden	4.4–15.4	Koch 1987	Koch et al. [1]
Sweden	18.4	mDDE	Jalevik et al. [26]
The Netherlands	9.7	Weerheijm 2001	Weerheijm et al. [68]
The Netherlands	14.25	MIH 2001	Jasulaityte et al. [69]
Turkey	14.9	EAPD 2003	Kuscu et al. [70]

Table 3.3 Overview of the prevalence studies on HSPM

Country	Prevalence (%)	Reference
Iraq	6.6	Ghanim et al. [46]
The Netherlands	4.9	Elfrink et al. [7]
The Netherlands	9.0	Elfrink et al. [72]

odds ratio (OR) for MIH was 5.3 (95 % CI: 2.9–9.4) and in children with severe HSPM, the OR was 4.0 (95 % CI: 2.6–6.3).

Clinical Implications

Opacities on second primary molars (HSPM) and erupting permanent incisors are potential indicators for MIH. While MIH cannot be confirmed until the complete eruption of all four first permanent molars the dental team should be alert for such lesions as soon as teeth erupt. In the case of the second primary molars, this is around 2 years of age. This emphasizes the importance of raising parental awareness of oral health and establishing a dental home early in their child's life. Understanding these lesions as predictors of MIH means that it is possible to inform patients of the potential implications and need for proactive prevention and dental management. More frequent dental checkups may be needed during the period of first permanent molar eruption [72]. When opacities on newly erupting first permanent molars are first identified, it is important to discuss the diagnosis of MIH not only because hypomineralized teeth cause discomfort and develop caries more easily but also because the permanent incisors may be affected. This can prepare the individual child and their parents for future esthetic issues that may become evident once the incisors erupt. However it is also equally important to reassure affected children and their parents that permanent teeth other than first molars and incisors are unlikely to be hypomineralized because the timing of development of the remainder of the permanent dentition does not coincide with that of the first molars and incisors.

Future Goals

In most countries where more than one prevalence study has been performed (see Tables 3.2 and 3.3), the more recent study shows a higher prevalence. It is unknown if this is an expression of increasing prevalence or an example of improved recognition of this particular dental enamel defect. Data from around the world and from different birth cohorts are important not only for future dental service planning but also in helping the search for better understanding of the etiological factors involved in MIH and HSPM. From that point of view it now seems advisable to incorporate assessment of MIH and HSPM prevalence figures with standardized score criteria into national epidemiological caries prevalence studies in order to answer the question as to whether the prevalence of MIH and HSPM is stable or whether it increases or decreases over time.

> **Conclusion**
>
> HSPM and MIH require early diagnosis. HSPM as well as demarcated opacities on erupting permanent incisors can be used as predictor for MIH though not exclusively. Children who experience one or more of the possible etiological factors need to be checked for HSPM and/or MIH. Children with HSPM or MIH need increased surveillance by the dental team including more frequent dental checkups and additional preventive advice particularly around the time of eruption of the second primary and first permanent molars. Prevention and treatment options for MIH and HSPM will be addressed further in Chaps. 8, 9, 10 and 11.

References

1. Koch G, Hallonsten AL, Ludvigsson N, Hansson BO, Holst A, Ullbro C. Epidemiologic study of idiopathic enamel hypomineralization in permanent teeth of Swedish children. Community Dent Oral Epidemiol. 1987;15(5):279–85.

2. Weerheijm KL. Molar incisor hypomineralisation (MIH). Eur J Paediatr Dent. 2003;4(3):114–20.
3. Weerheijm KL, Jalevik B, Alaluusua S. Molar-incisor hypomineralisation. Caries Res. 2001;35(5):390–1.
4. Weerheijm KL, Duggal M, Mejare I, Papagiannoulis L, Koch G, Martens LC, et al. Judgement criteria for molar incisor hypomineralisation (MIH) in epidemiologic studies: a summary of the European meeting on MIH held in Athens. Eur J Paediatr Dent. 2003;4(3):110–3.
5. Elfrink M. Deciduous molar hypomineralisation, its nature and nurture. Thesis. Amsterdam: University of Amsterdam (UvA); 2012. p. 1–160.
6. Jalevik B. Prevalence and diagnosis of molar-incisor- hypomineralisation (MIH): a systematic review. Eur Arch Paediatr Dent. 2010;11(2):59–64.
7. Elfrink ME, Schuller AA, Weerheijm KL, Veerkamp JS. Hypomineralized second primary molars: prevalence data in Dutch 5-year-olds. Caries Res. 2008;42(4):282–5.
8. Elfrink ME, Schuller AA, Veerkamp JS, Poorterman JH, Moll HA, ten Cate BJ. Factors increasing the caries risk of second primary molars in 5-year-old Dutch children. Int J Paediatr Dent. 2010;20(2):151–7.
9. Oliver K, Messer LB, Manton DJ, Kan K, Ng F, Olsen C, et al. Distribution and severity of molar hypomineralisation: trial of a new severity index. Int J Paediatr Dent. 2014;24(2):131–51. doi:10.1111/ipd.12040. Epub 2013 May 22.
10. Malmgren B, Andreasen J, Flores M, Robertson A, DiAngelis A, Andersson L, et al. International association of dental traumatology guidelines for the management of traumatic dental injuries: 3 injuries in the primary dentition. Dent Traumatol. 2012;28(3):174–82.
11. Jalevik B, Klingberg G. Treatment outcomes and dental anxiety in 18-year-olds with MIH, comparisons with healthy controls – a longitudinal study. Int J Paediatr Dent. 2012;22(2):85–91.
12. Suga S. Enamel hypomineralization viewed from the pattern of progressive mineralization of human and monkey developing enamel. Adv Dent Res. 1989;3(2):188–98.
13. Suckling GW. Developmental defects of enamel–historical and present-day perspectives of their pathogenesis. Adv Dent Res. 1989;3(2):87–94.
14. Fagrell TG, Ludvigsson J, Ullbro C, Lundin SA, Koch G. Aetiology of severe demarcated enamel opacities–an evaluation based on prospective medical and social data from 17,000 children. Swed Dent J. 2011;35(2):57–67.
15. Fagrell TG, Salmon P, Melin L, Noren JG. Onset of molar incisor hypomineralization (MIH). Swed Dent J. 2013;37(2):61–70.
16. Lygidakis NA, Dimou G, Briseniou E. Molar-incisor-hypomineralisation (MIH). Retrospective clinical study in Greek children. I. Prevalence and defect characteristics. Eur Arch Paediatr Dent. 2008;9(4):200–6.
17. Whatling R, Fearne JM. Molar incisor hypomineralization: a study of aetiological factors in a group of UK children. Int J Paediatr Dent. 2008;18(3):155–62.
18. Alaluusua S. Aetiology of molar-incisor-hypomineralisation: a systematic review. Eur Arch Paediatr Dent. 2010;11(2):53–8.
19. Jontell M, Linde A. Nutritional aspects on tooth formation. World Rev Nutr Diet. 1986;48:114–36.
20. van Amerongen WE, Kreulen CM. Cheese molars: a pilot study of the etiology of hypocalcifications in first permanent molars. J Dent Child. 1995;62(4):266–9.
21. Beentjes VE, Weerheijm KL, Groen HJ. Factors involved in the aetiology of molar-incisor hypomineralisation (MIH). Eur J Paediatr Dent. 2002;3(1):9–13.
22. Fearne JM, Bryan EM, Elliman AM, Brook AH, Williams DM. Enamel defects in the primary dentition of children born weighing less than 2000 g. Br Dent J. 1990;168(11):433–7.
23. Seow WK. A study of the development of the permanent dentition in very low birthweight children. Pediatr Dent. 1996;18(5):379–84.
24. Aine L, Backstrom MC, Maki R, Kuusela AL, Koivisto AM, Ikonen RS, et al. Enamel defects in primary and permanent teeth of children born prematurely. J Oral Pathol Med. 2000;29(8):403–9.

25. Crombie F, Manton D, Kilpatrick N. Aetiology of molar-incisor hypomineralization: a critical review. Int J Paediatr Dent. 2009;19(2):73–83.
26. Jalevik B, Klingberg G, Barregard L, Noren JG. The prevalence of demarcated opacities in permanent first molars in a group of Swedish children. Acta Odontol Scand. 2001;59(5):255–60.
27. Alaluusua S, Lukinmaa PL, Koskimies M, Pirinen S, Holtta P, Kallio M, et al. Developmental dental defects associated with long breast feeding. Eur J Oral Sci. 1996;104(5–6):493–7.
28. Alaluusua S, Calderara P, Gerthoux PM, Lukinmaa PL, Kovero O, Needham L, et al. Developmental dental aberrations after the dioxin accident in Seveso. Environ Health Perspect. 2004;112(13):1313–8.
29. Alaluusua S, Lukinmaa PL, Torppa J, Tuomisto J, Vartiainen T. Developing teeth as biomarker of dioxin exposure. Lancet. 1999;353(9148):206.
30. Alaluusua S, Lukinmaa PL, Vartiainen T, Partanen AM, Torppa J, Tuomisto J. Polychlorinated dibenzo-p-dioxins and dibenzofurans via mother's milk may cause developmental defects in the child's teeth. Environ Toxicol Pharmacol. 1996;1:193–7.
31. Holtta P, Kiviranta H, Leppaniemi A, Vartiainen T, Lukinmaa PL, Alaluusua S. Developmental dental defects in children who reside by a river polluted by dioxins and furans. Arch Environ Health. 2001;56(6):522–8.
32. Jedeon K, De la Dure-Molla M, Brookes SJ, Loiodice S, Marciano C, Kirkham J, et al. Enamel defects reflect perinatal exposure to bisphenol A. Am J Pathol. 2013;183(1):108–18.
33. Kuscu OO, Caglar E, Aslan S, Durmusoglu E, Karademir A, Sandalli N. The prevalence of molar incisor hypomineralization (MIH) in a group of children in a highly polluted urban region and a windfarm-green energy island. Int J Paediatr Dent. 2009;19(3):176–85.
34. Laisi S, Kiviranta H, Lukinmaa PL, Vartiainen T, Alaluusua S. Molar-incisor-hypomineralisation and dioxins: new findings. Eur Arch Paediatr Dent. 2008;9(4):224–7.
35. Salmela E, Lukinmaa PL, Partanen AM, Sahlberg C, Alaluusua S. Combined effect of fluoride and 2,3,7,8-tetrachlorodibenzo-p-dioxin on mouse dental hard tissue formation in vitro. Arch Toxicol. 2011;85(8):953–63.
36. Jalevik B, Noren JG. Enamel hypomineralization of permanent first molars: a morphological study and survey of possible aetiological factors. Int J Paediatr Dent. 2000;10(4):278–89.
37. van Amerongen WE, Kreulen CM. Cheese molars: a pilot study of the etiology of hypocalci-fications in first permanent molars. ASDC J Dent Child. 1995;62(4):266–9.
38. Tung K, Fujita H, Yamashita Y, Takagi Y. Effect of turpentine-induced fever during the enamel formation of rat incisor. Arch Oral Biol. 2006;51(6):464–70.
39. Laisi S, Ess A, Sahlberg C, Arvio P, Lukinmaa PL, Alaluusua S. Amoxicillin may cause molar incisor hypomineralization. J Dent Res. 2009;88(2):132–6.
40. Sahlberg C, Pavlic A, Ess A, Lukinmaa PL, Salmela E, Alaluusua S. Combined effect of amoxicillin and sodium fluoride on the structure of developing mouse enamel in vitro. Arch Oral Biol. 2013;58(9):1155–64.
41. Kumazawa K, Sawada T, Yanagisawa T, Shintani S. Effect of single-dose amoxicillin on rat incisor odontogenesis: a morphological study. Clin Oral Investig. 2012;16(3):835–42.
42. Wogelius P, Haubek D, Poulsen S. Prevalence and distribution of demarcated opacities in permanent 1st molars and incisors in 6 to 8-year-old Danish children. Acta Odontol Scand. 2008;66(1):58–64.
43. Sahlstrand P, Lith A, Hakeberg M, Noren JG. Timing of mineralization of homologues perma-nent teeth–an evaluation of the dental maturation in panoramic radiographs. Swed Dent J. 2013;37(3):111–9.
44. Brook AH, Smith JM. The aetiology of developmental defects of enamel: a prevalence and family study in East London, U.K. Connect Tissue Res. 1998;39(1–3):151–6.
45. Jeremias F, Koruyucu M, Kuchler EC, Bayram M, Tuna EB, Deeley K, et al. Genes expressed in dental enamel development are associated with molar-incisor hypomineralization. Arch Oral Biol. 2013;58(10):1434–42.
46. Ghanim AM, Morgan MV, Marino RJ, Bailey DL, Manton DJ. Risk factors of hypominer-alised second primary molars in a group of Iraqi schoolchildren. Eur Arch Paediatr Dent. 2012;13(3):111–8.

47. Elfrink ME et al. Pre- and postnatal determinants of deciduous molar hypomineralisation in 6-year-old children. The generation R study. PLoS One. 2014;9(7):e91057. doi:10.1371/journal.pone.0091057 eCollection 2014.
48. Elfrink M, Moll H, Kiefte-de Jong J, El Marroun H, Jaddoe V, Hofman A, et al. Is maternal use of medicines during pregnancy associated with deciduous molar hypomineralisation in the offspring? A prospective, population-based study. Drug Saf. 2013;36(8):627–33.
49. Arrow P. Prevalence of developmental enamel defects of the first permanent molars among school children in Western Australia. Aust Dent J. 2008;53(3):250–9.
50. Balmer RC, Laskey D, Mahoney E, Toumba KJ. Prevalence of enamel defects and MIH in non-fluoridated and fluoridated communities. Eur J Paediatr Dent. 2005;6(4):209–12.
51. Muratbegovic A, Markovic N, Ganibegovic SM. Molar incisor hypomineralisation in Bosnia and Herzegovina: aetiology and clinical consequences in medium caries activity population. Eur Arch Paediatr Dent. 2007;8(4):189–94.
52. Soviero V, Haubek D, Trindade C, Da Matta T, Poulsen S. Prevalence and distribution of demarcated opacities and their sequelae in permanent 1st molars and incisors in 7 to 13-year-old Brazilian children. Acta Odontol Scand. 2009;67(3):170–5.
53. da Costa-Silva CM, Jeremias F, de Souza JF, Cordeiro Rde C, Santos-Pinto L, Zuanon AC. Molar incisor hypomineralization: prevalence, severity and clinical consequences in Brazilian children. Int J Paediatr Dent. 2010;20(6):426–34.
54. Cho SY, Ki Y, Chu V. Molar incisor hypomineralization in Hong Kong Chinese children. Int J Paediatr Dent. 2008;18(5):348–52.
55. Leppaniemi A, Lukinmaa PL, Alaluusua S. Nonfluoride hypomineralizations in the permanent first molars and their impact on the treatment need. Caries Res. 2001;35(1):36–40.
56. Petrou MA, Giraki M, Bissar AR, Basner R, Wempe C, Altarabulsi M, et al. Prevalence of molar-incisor-hypomineralisation among school children in four German cities. Int J Paediatr Dent. 2013. doi:10.1111/ipd.12089. Epub ahead of print.
57. Parikh DR, Ganesh M, Bhaskar V. Prevalence and characteristics of molar incisor hypomineralisation (MIH) in the child population residing in Gandhinagar, Gujarat, India. Eur Arch Paediatr Dent. 2012;13(1):21–6.
58. Ghanim A, Bagheri R, Golkari A, Manton D. Molar-incisor hypomineralisation: a prevalence study amongst primary schoolchildren of Shiraz, Iran. Eur Arch Paediatr Dent. 2014;15(2):75–82. doi:10.1007/s40368-013-0067-y. Epub 2013 Jul 17.
59. Ghanim A, Morgan M, Marino R, Bailey D, Manton D. Molar-incisor hypomineralisation: prevalence and defect characteristics in Iraqi children. Int J Paediatr Dent. 2011;21(6):413–21.
60. Calderara PC, Gerthoux PM, Mocarelli P, Lukinmaa PL, Tramacere PL, Alaluusua S. The prevalence of molar incisor hypomineralisation (MIH) in a group of Italian school children. Eur J Paediatr Dent. 2005;6(2):79–83.
61. Zawaideh FI, Al-Jundi SH, Al-Jaljoli MH. Molar incisor hypomineralisation: prevalence in Jordanian children and clinical characteristics. Eur Arch Paediatr Dent. 2011;12(1):31–6.
62. Fteita D, Ali A, Alaluusua S. Molar-incisor hypomineralization (MIH) in a group of school-aged children in Benghazi, Libya. Eur Arch Paediatr Dent. 2006;7(2):92–5.
63. Jasulaityte L, Veerkamp JS, Weerheijm KL. Molar incisor hypomineralization: review and prevalence data from the study of primary school children in Kaunas/Lithuania. Eur Arch Paediatr Dent. 2007;8(2):87–94.
64. Mahoney EK, Morrison DG. The prevalence of molar-incisor hypomineralisation (MIH) in Wainuiomata children. N Z Dent J. 2009;105(4):121–7.
65. Mahoney EK, Morrison DG. Further examination of the prevalence of MIH in the Wellington region. N Z Dent J. 2011;107(3):79–84.
66. Martinez Gomez TP, Guinot Jimeno F, Bellet Dalmau LJ, Giner TL. Prevalence of molar-incisor hypomineralisation observed using transillumination in a group of children from Barcelona (Spain). Int J Paediatr Dent. 2012;22(2):100–9.
67. Garcia-Margarit M, Catala-Pizarro M, Montiel-Company JM, Almerich-Silla JM. Epidemiologic study of molar-incisor hypomineralization in 8-year-old Spanish children. Int J Paediatr Dent. 2014;24(1):14–22. doi:10.1111/ipd.12020. Epub 2013 Jan 14.

68. Weerheijm KL, Groen HJ, Beentjes VE, Poorterman JH. Prevalence of cheese molars in eleven-year-old Dutch children. ASDC J Dent Child. 2001;68(4):259–62. 29.
69. Jasulaityte L, Weerheijm KL, Veerkamp JS. Prevalence of molar-incisor-hypomineralisation among children participating in the Dutch National Epidemiological Survey (2003). Eur Arch Paediatr Dent. 2008;9(4):218–23.
70. Kuscu OO, Caglar E, Sandalli N. The prevalence and aetiology of molar-incisor hypomineralisation in a group of children in Istanbul. Eur J Paediatr Dent. 2008;9(3):139–44.
71. Chawla N, Messer LB, Silva M. Clinical studies on molar-incisor-hypomineralisation part 1: distribution and putative associations. Eur Arch Paediatr Dent. 2008;9(4):180–90.
72. Elfrink ME, ten Cate JM, Jaddoe VW, Hofman A, Moll HA, Veerkamp JS. Deciduous molar hypomineralization and molar incisor hypomineralization. J Dent Res. 2012;91(6):551–5.

Syndromes and Diseases Associated with Developmental Defects of Enamel

4

Mike Harrison, Angus Cameron, and Nicky Kilpatrick

Abstract

Some patients have what may be described as "syndromic teeth." The size, number or crown/root morphology can indicate that the patient is affected by a recognized malformation syndrome. Developmental defects of enamel (DDE) can sometimes be part of a constellation of developmental changes elsewhere in the body and may even provide diagnostic clues. If the underlying condition includes processes that may affect enamel formation in more generalized, non-genetic ways, it can be difficult to be precise about the mechanism of the defect. Examples include renal disease and congenital cardiac defects, both of which can be of genetic origin and disturb enamel formation by genetic and/or pathological means. This section will describe some diseases and syndromes reported to exhibit DDE, with some guidance about whether they are likely to have direct or indirect association.

Introduction

As is discussed in other chapters (Chaps. 1, 2 and 5), developmental defects of enamel (DDE) have been reported to occur in association with a wide range of systemic conditions. For convenience this chapter is divided into diseases and

M. Harrison, BDS, MScD, MPhil (✉)
Department of Pediatric Dentistry, Guy's and St Thomas' Dental Institute,
Floor 22 Guys Tower, Great Maze Pond, London SE1 9RT, UK
e-mail: mike.harrison1@nhs.net

A. Cameron, BDS, MDSc
Department of Pediatric Dentistry, Westmead Hospital and The University of Sydney,
Darcy Rd, Westmead, NSW 2145, Australia
e-mail: Angus.Cameron@health.nsw.gov.au

N. Kilpatrick, BDS, PhD
Cleft and Craniofacial Research, Murdoch Childrens Research Institute,
Flemington Road, Parkville, Melbourne, VIC 3052, Australia
e-mail: nicky@bassdata.com.au

© Springer-Verlag Berlin Heidelberg 2015
B.K. Drummond, N. Kilpatrick (eds.), *Planning and Care for Children and Adolescents with Dental Enamel Defects: Etiology, Research and Contemporary Management*, DOI 10.1007/978-3-662-44800-7_4

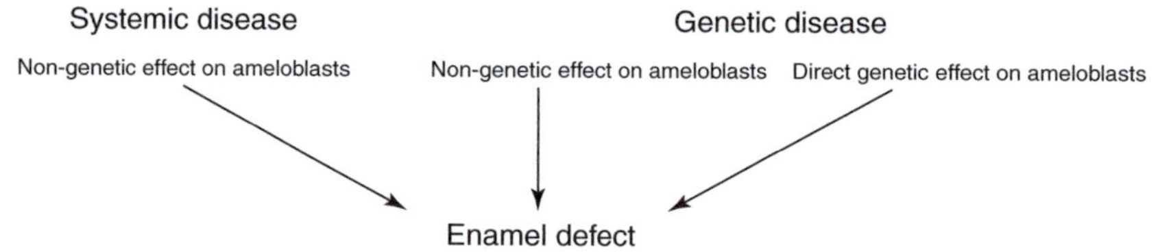

Fig. 4.1 Classification of the etiology of enamel defects in relation to systemic diseases or genetic syndromes

syndromes, but in reality there is much overlap with many systemic diseases having an identified genetic origin e.g. cystic fibrosis.

These disorders of enamel will be considered in three ways (see Fig. 4.1):

(i) Those presenting with systemic disease as a pathological but non-genetic effect on ameloblasts
(ii) Those presenting with a genetic disease and with a similar pathological but non-genetic effect on the ameloblasts
(iii) Those specific genetic diseases in which the affected gene is known to be directly involved in amelogenesis

It is important to distinguish between the terms hypoplasia and hypomineralization in the diagnosis of enamel defects. Hypoplasia is a defect in the quantity of the enamel. It results from a disorder of amelogenesis during the appositional or initial secretory stage of enamel formation. It may appear as thinner enamel, pits, or grooves. Adjacent enamel may also be hypomineralized. Hypomineralization relates to a deficiency in the quality of the enamel, presenting primarily as an opacity (or porosity) in the enamel. This may be present superficially or through the full thickness of the enamel. Most hypomineralization defects occur during the later maturation phases of tooth development.

Systemic Disease with a Non-genetic Effect on Ameloblasts

Preterm and Low Birth Weight Infants

It is not uncommon for infants to be born as early as 25 weeks gestation and not only to survive, but develop with relatively few physical or intellectual consequences. However the stigmata of the preterm infant can manifest even in children born up to 36 weeks, related to conditions including perinatal respiratory distress, intracranial bleeds, pulmonary immaturity, persistent ductus arteriosus and ventricular septal foramina, necrotizing enterocolitis and some debilitating infections. Long-term ventilation via oral or nasal intubation, hyperbilirubinemia leading to jaundice and suboptimal nutrition all contribute to the comorbidity. Neonatal hypocalcemia presents in all newborn infants up to 48 h until the development of normal calcitonin and parathyroid hormone levels. However this hypocalcemia is often more severe in preterm neonates resulting in altered calcification of the enamel matrix.

The timing of development of the primary and permanent dentitions means that amelogenesis in the primary dentition is particularly vulnerable to disturbances as a consequence of prematurity. Thus, in the primary dentition, there is a direct association between low birth weight (<1,500 g) and both enamel opacities and hypoplasia [1].

Although the actual process of mineralization of permanent dentition enamel does not commence until around the time of a full-term birth, some studies have reported an increased risk of enamel defects in the first permanent molars [2–4]. However, the strength of the evidence to support a causal relationship between preterm birth and DDE in the permanent dentition remains limited at this time [1].

Renal Disease

Renal function is essential in homeostatic regulation of the calcium and phosphate salts needed for the formation of all mineralized tissues. Although odontogenesis is notably different from osteogenesis its processes are equally susceptible to dysregulation of mineralization resulting from renal failure. Hypoplastic horizontal enamel defects are characteristic of acute renal disease in early childhood. The position of the defects on the crowns of the permanent teeth is often strikingly coincident with the age of the child at the onset of disease. Normal full-thickness enamel formation will be seen following remission or resolution of the acute phase.

Nephrotic Syndrome

Nephrotic syndrome is a non-specific kidney disorder associated with damage to the glomeruli which alters their capacity to filter substances transported in the blood. Despite the term "syndrome" this is a heterogeneous range of conditions whose genetic basis is currently not fully understood. It has been reported to cause hypomineralization defects [5] though the mechanism is somewhat unclear. A failure of the highly selective filtration in the glomerulus leads to heavy loss of albumin, lipids and other proteins. Widespread edema is the initial feature but loss of macromolecules and binding proteins leads to significant morbidity and even mortality. The primary cause of this edema is failure of water and salt excretion and it must be presumed that this also disrupts calcium and phosphate homeostasis, resulting in defects in tissues which are undergoing mineralization.

Celiac Disease

Enamel defects occur with varying severity in patients with celiac disease, an immune-mediated disorder in which damage to the mucosa of the small intestine

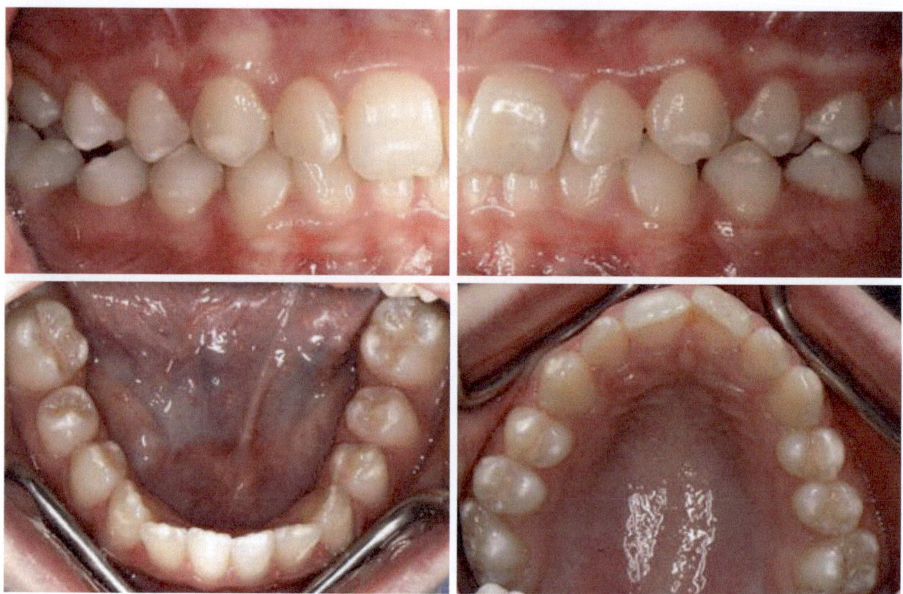

Fig. 4.2 Grade I enamel defects in a 14-year-old girl diagnosed with celiac disease at the age of 9 years (Courtesy of Dr AK Natarajan, New Zealand)

occurs causing malabsorption when susceptible individuals ingest proline- and glutamine-rich proteins ("gluten") in wheat, rye, and barley [6]. The risk of enamel defects has been reported to be higher with the presence of HLA-DR52–53 and DQ7, human leukocyte antigens [7]. The prevalence has been reported in the primary dentition as between 5.8 and 13.3 % and in the permanent dentition between 9.5 and 95 % with incisors being the most commonly affected teeth [8–11]. This is not unexpected as the crowns of the incisors form in the first year of life when gluten is first introduced into the diet. The severity of the defects is related to the length of time of gluten exposure before the condition is diagnosed. Once gluten is removed from the diet, symptoms will disappear but enamel defects will remain. The classification of enamel defects in celiac disease is usually that reported by Aine in 1986; Grade 0 exhibits no defects; Grade I exhibits a color defect with cream, yellow, or brown opacities; Grade II exhibits rough enamel surface with shallow horizontal grooves or pits and may include opacities and discoloration; Grade III exhibits structural defects, a rough surface, deep horizontal grooves, vertical pits and large discolored opacities; and Grade IV exhibits severe structural defects with pointed cusp tips and/or thinned uneven incisal edges. Usually defects can be detected in a pattern across all four quadrants. Figure 4.2 shows a typical pattern of Grade I enamel defects in a 14-year-old female diagnosed with celiac disease at 9 years of age.

There are two possible mechanisms underpinning the DDE lesions seen in celiac disease; one relates to malabsorption leading to hypocalcemia, while the other suggests that there may be an immune response to the ameloblasts [12]. Irrespective of the mechanism, the pattern of the DDE should always be recorded carefully by clinicians in all patients who have a diagnosis of celiac disease. Conversely when a

Fig. 4.3 (**a**) Shows the clinical image and (**b**) radiograph of a 10-year-old treated with chemotherapy and radiotherapy for a hepatoblastoma age 2 years

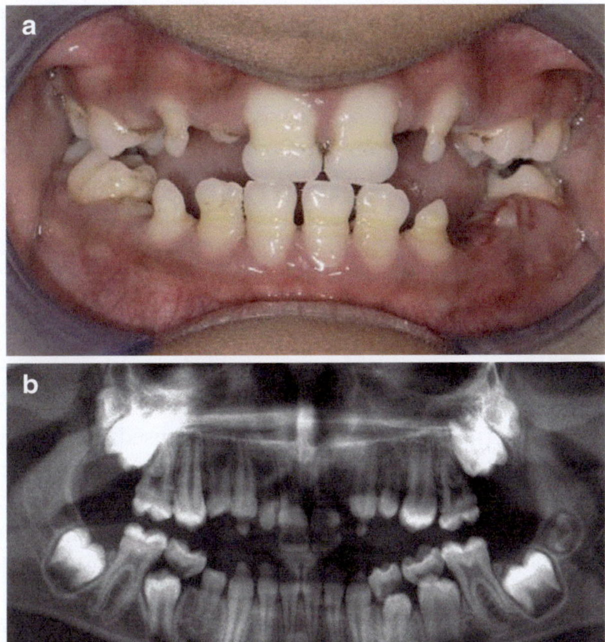

pattern of specific enamel defects occurs and no other cause can be determined, clinicians should consider celiac disease in the differential diagnosis. Questions in the history should include occurrence of recurrent aphthous ulceration, abdominal pain, diarrhea, poor weight gain, fatigue, anemia or a family history of celiac disease. A referral should be made to a pediatrician or gastroenterologist for testing with a description of the oral signs that have been detected.

Childhood Oncology

The enamel organ is very sensitive to the toxic effects of chemotherapeutic agents and radiation therapy. The effects of radiation may be attributable to both deterministic effects (non-stochastic, dose dependent) and stochastic effects (random, no minimum dose). Agenesis, microdontia, and ridges of hypoplasia may be seen, almost always with concomitant disturbances of dentin development and root malformations in particular (Fig. 4.3a, b).

The leukemias are the most common group of childhood malignancies; thus the effects of therapy on amelogenesis tend to be generalized. Therapy for solid tumors such as brain and ocular lesions is often more targeted and more likely to affect one side or even one quadrant. The severity of the defects will be determined primarily by the age of the child when therapy is commenced and then by the type, intensity and duration of therapy [13].

Genetic Systemic Disease with an Indirect Effect on Amelogenesis

The processes of odontogenesis, including amelogenesis, are dependent on complex temporal and spatial interaction between genes and gene products, the contemporary understanding of which is less than comprehensive. While this section summarizes some monogenic diseases where the causative gene is currently not thought to be involved in amelogenesis, there may be a future time when a direct cause-and-effect model is identified.

Rickets

The term "rickets" has been traditionally used to describe the skeletal disease associated with deficiency in vitamin D, be that a dietary deficiency or one resulting from insufficient exposure to sunlight. However more recently the term has been expanded to include inherited metabolic bone diseases causing defects in mineral metabolism. Advances in understanding the molecular basis of disorders of hard tissue formation and regulation have led to discovery of specific genes and their protein products which, when mutated, lead to specific bone diseases. As is often the case, where skeletal bone metabolism is defective, odontogenesis is affected in some way [14].

Vitamin D-Dependent Rickets (VDDR)

Deficiency of vitamin D and calcium was a very common cause of rickets in the past. However it almost disappeared in the Western world during the early twentieth century thanks to the fortification of foods with vitamin D. More recently there has been a resurgence in the prevalence of VDDR which has been linked to inadequate exposure to sunlight. The factors behind this remain putative but include heightened awareness of the risk of skin cancer, cultural clothing practices leading to women being fully covered and dark-skinned people living in northern (cloudy) climates with little daily sunlight.

Enamel and dentin defects have long been reported in VDDR, with hypoplastic (often discolored) enamel, large pulp chambers, short roots and interglobular dentin spaces [15]. These defects are closely linked to circulating levels of the active metabolic form of vitamin D, namely 1,25-dihydroxyvitamin D_3. Direct effects on the enamel organ and odontoblasts can cause defects in both matrix secretion and mineralization resulting in hypoplastic enamel which may also be hypomineralized (Fig. 4.4). Importantly early diagnosis of VDDR and appropriate dietary supplementation can improve both skeletal and dental mineralization.

X-Linked Hypophosphatemic Rickets (XLHR)

While rare, XLHR is the most common cause of familial rickets with an incidence of 1:20,000 births [16]. The disease is related to an isolated phosphate

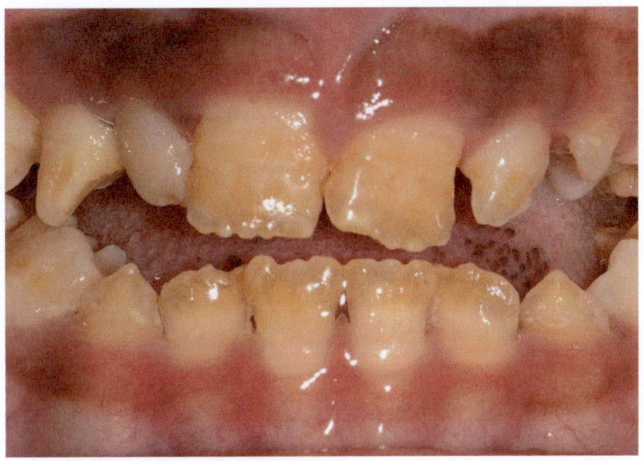

Fig. 4.4 Vitamin D-dependent rickets showing hypoplastic enamel defects

transport defect caused by mutations in the *PHEX* gene that results in increased inhibition of both skeletal and dental mineralization. This X-linked dominantly inherited condition is characterized clinically by hypophosphatemia (reduced phosphate level in the blood), growth retardation, rickets and well-recognized dental manifestations. Initial descriptions of XLHR emphasized the poor clinical response to vitamin D rather than the distinctive finding of marked hypophosphatemia, hence the historical use of the term "vitamin D-resistant rickets."

As with some other familial forms of rickets, XLHR is associated with spontaneous dental abscesses which are probably associated with the thin, hypomineralized dentin and large pulp chambers. The enamel in these conditions often appears macroscopically normal though enamel hypoplasia, cracks and defects have been reported [17]. The mechanism behind these enamel defects, which are reported to occur in up to 28 % of XLHR affected individuals [18], is currently unclear; however they may well contribute to the apparently spontaneous nature of these abscesses (Fig. 4.5a, b). The dental manifestations can be particularly miserable for the affected individuals and are also difficult to manage clinically [19]. Early clinical and molecular diagnosis of these familial disorders may lead to timely correction of the metabolic defect. While medical management, aimed at controlling serum calcium and phosphate, undoubtedly has a positive effect on skeletal development, there is also evidence that the associated dental defects may be partially or totally rescued [20].

Cystic Fibrosis

Cystic fibrosis (CF) is a chronic respiratory disease with associated gastrointestinal disease, exocrine pancreatic insufficiency and delayed growth. It is caused by mutations in the cystic fibrosis transmembrane regulator protein (*CFTR*). Skeletal and dental developmental delays are known comorbidities in CF and the incidence of hypoplastic enamel defects has been reported to be higher than

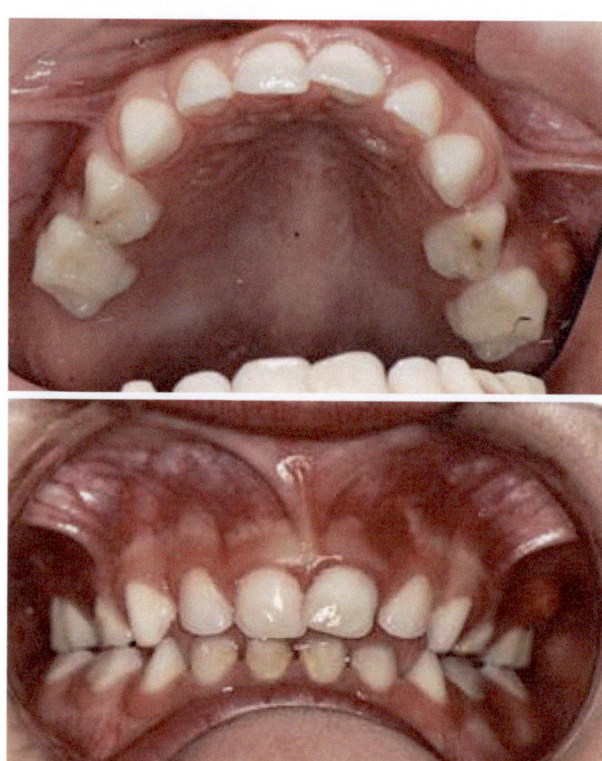

Fig. 4.5 Show the relatively normal macroscopic appearance of the primary dentition of a child with X-linked hypophosphatemic rickets. Note the abscess associated with the non-carious upper left second primary molar

in the normal population [21, 22]. Currently the exact mechanism behind the occurrence of DDE in CF is unknown, and as such these defects may simply represent those expected in any debilitating illness of early childhood. However *CFTR* is known to regulate the carbonic acid buffer system, controlling the pH critical for ameloblast function and apatite deposition [23] and therefore it is possible that there is some direct genetic impact on enamel formation yet to be identified.

Tuberous Sclerosis (TS)

TS is a genetic disorder that can affect multiple organ systems with benign hamartomas. It is considered a common epilepsy syndrome and may be associated with autism spectrum disorder and other neurocognitive disabilities. It has long been recognized that enamel pits (hypoplasia) are a variable feature of TS. These pits may be widespread, mimicking some pitted forms of amelogenesis imperfecta (AI), or sparse with fewer than 10 pits in an entire dentition (Fig. 4.6). There is

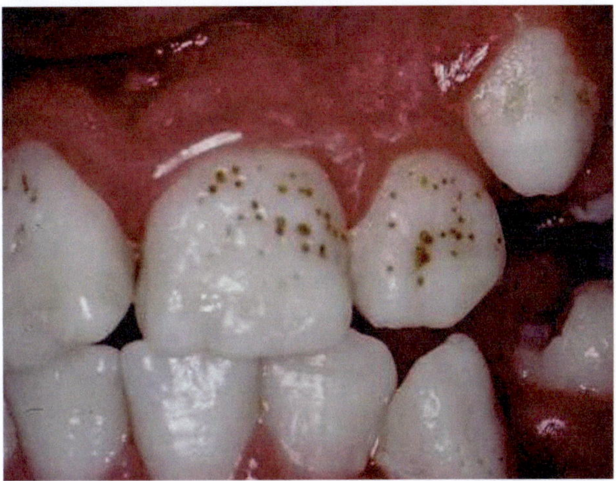

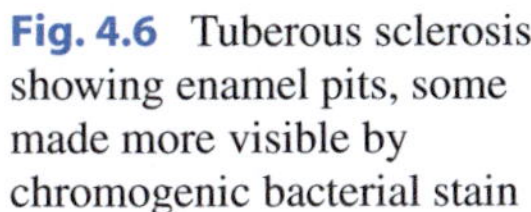

Fig. 4.6 Tuberous sclerosis, showing enamel pits, some made more visible by chromogenic bacterial stain

debate as to whether the presence of enamel pits in first-degree relatives of individuals with TS is a sign of asymptomatic carrier status. Screening for the presence of enamel pits in TS relatives is not however yet considered a reliable method of diagnosis [24].

Other Syndromes with Enamel Defects

The Online Mendelian Inheritance in Man (OMIM) database is a catalogue of several thousand human malformation syndromes [25]. A search for "enamel defects" among these generates a considerable number of positive results. Many of these syndromes are extremely rare. Reports of dental manifestations associated with these syndromes are even more uncommon and potentially unreliable as the dental phenotype is rarely reported by a dentist. One example of a syndrome reportedly associated with DDE is Usher syndrome in which hypoplastic enamel has been described in a very small number of cases [26]. However it is important to treat with circumspection reports of enamel defects being associated with specific rare syndromes, unless the numbers are sufficient to support a true association. Furthermore in syndromes where systemic illness or failure to thrive are features of early childhood, the enamel defects may be secondary to the illness and any association with the syndrome itself may be spurious.

The increased reported incidence of enamel defects in 22q11.2 deletion syndrome (velocardiofacial syndrome) is a good example of a positive association having being demonstrated in a large cohort study including a comprehensive dental examination [27]. Although affected children can variously demonstrate hypocalcemia and/or hypoparathyroidism, congenital cardiac anomalies and premature birth, this study found the presence of enamel hypoplasia and hypomineralization defects to be independent of the primary disorder.

Syndromes with Direct Genetic Effect on Ameloblasts

There are very few truly syndromic AI conditions and equally few monogenic disorders with proven influence on amelogenesis. Those listed below are far from an exhaustive list, but it is likely that many syndromes reported to express enamel defects as part of the phenotype will in time reveal an expanded family of genes directly involved in amelogenesis.

Tricho-Dento-Osseous Syndrome (TDO)

TDO manifests as kinky hair shafts, thin hypoplastic enamel, and increased thickness of cranial bones. Abscess formation is common due to the morphology of the taurodontic pulp chambers and extended pulp horns combined with rapid attrition of the enamel (Fig. 4.7). The responsible gene for TDO has been identified as *DLX3*, a homeobox gene expressed in all three affected tissues. A causative explanation of the pathogenesis of the hypoplastic enamel defect appears in a report by Nieminen and coworkers [28] explaining how the *DLX3* expression pattern fits with the finding that the principal dental tissue affected in TDO is the epithelially derived enamel.

RAS/MAPK Pathway Syndromes (Noonan, Costello, LEOPARD, and Cardio-Facio-Cutaneous Syndromes)

Recently it has been established that abnormal RAS signaling does actually have a negative effect on enamel formation in animal and human subjects with Costello syndrome [29]. Disorders with mutations in the molecules of the combined RAS/MAPK pathways lead to a number of other recognizable malformation

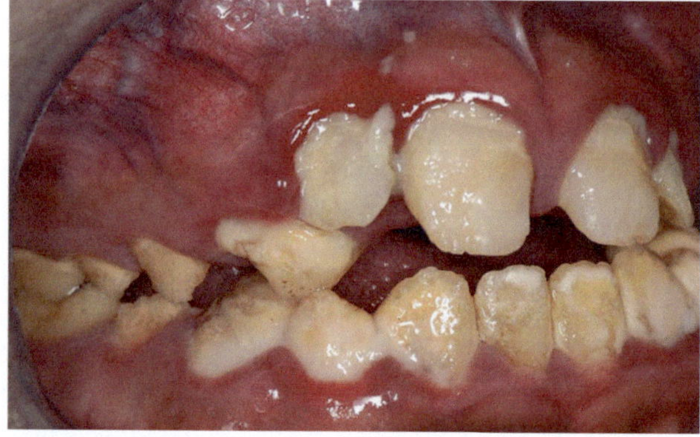

Fig. 4.7 Tricho-dento-osseous syndrome, showing thin hypoplastic enamel defects with some mild discoloration. Tooth sensitivity has resulted in extremely poor oral hygiene

syndromes, notably Noonan, LEOPARD, and cardio-facio-cutaneous syndromes. While hypoplastic enamel defects in these related conditions may be secondary to their associated syndromic cardiac anomalies, it may, in future, be possible to establish a direct developmental cause.

Enamel-Renal Syndrome/Enamel-Renal-Gingival Syndrome

Hunter and others reported nephrocalcinosis associated with AI and postulated that a clinical presentation of AI should prompt referral for renal ultrasound [30]. Subsequent similar reports were termed enamel-renal syndrome and it is now accepted that a small cohort of patients with hypoplastic, hypomineralized AI with multiple unerupted teeth may develop nephrocalcinosis. Furthermore, a clinically related group of AI patients with gingival fibromatosis have been found to have causative mutations in the *FAM20A* gene [31] (see Chap. 5).

Epidermolysis Bullosa (EB)

These conditions are characterized by severe fragility and blistering of the skin following minimal lateral pressure or trauma. Clinical types of EB are described by the level of tissue separation within the epidermis (EB simplex), basement membrane (junctional EB) and underlying connective tissue (dystrophic EB). The latter types, junctional and dystrophic EB, are associated with enamel defects ranging from thin hypoplasia through to widespread pitting or furrowing (Fig. 4.8a, b). A higher incidence of caries is noted in these groups [32] though this is also likely to be linked to the difficulties in maintaining oral hygiene when the oral mucosa is prone to blistering (Fig. 4.8c).

Autosomal Recessive Cone-Rod Dystrophy and Amelogenesis Imperfecta (Jalili Syndrome)

This is an extremely rare autosomal recessive form of severe hypomineralization AI in combination with reduced visual acuity, color vision abnormalities, photophobia and visual field loss. The causative gene has been identified as *CNNM4*, a gene involved in metal transportation. Interestingly, the clinical and radiographic appearances of the enamel are similar to those seen in AI resulting from mutations in a matrix metallopeptidase gene *MMP20*. Specialized metal transport is necessary in the phototransduction cascade in the retina, where *CNNM4* is also shown to play a role [33]. This monogenic condition demonstrates how mutations in a single gene expressed in development or regulation of different tissues can cause explainable dysplasia or dysfunction in each.

Fig. 4.8 (**a**) Localized thin enamel hypoplasia of the primary incisors in a child with junctional EB. (**b**) A primary molar from a child with EB showing characteristic pitted enamel and bizarre cusp morphology. (**c**) The characteristic intraoral bullae seen in a child with junctional EB which can hamper effective oral hygiene

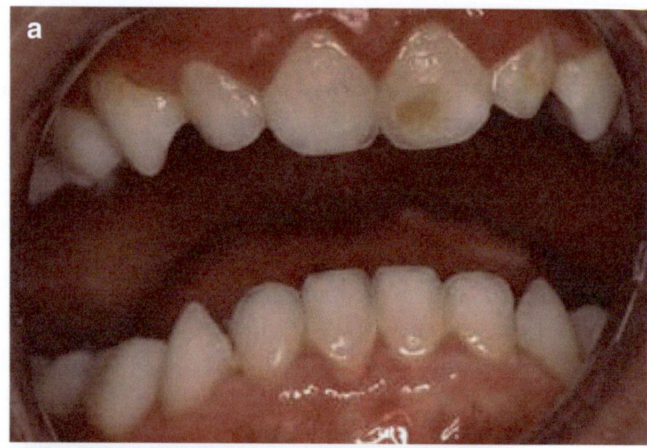

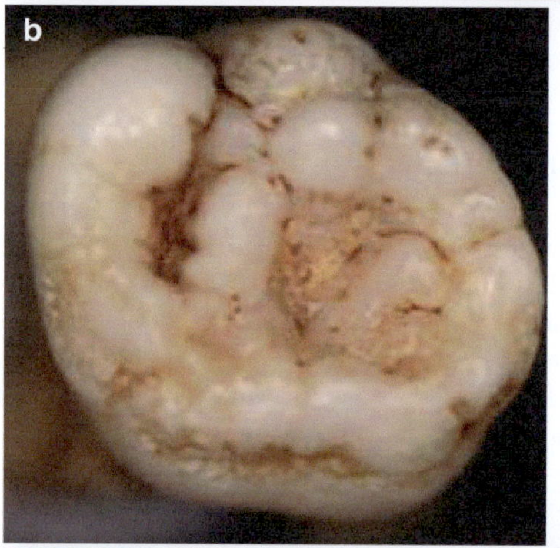

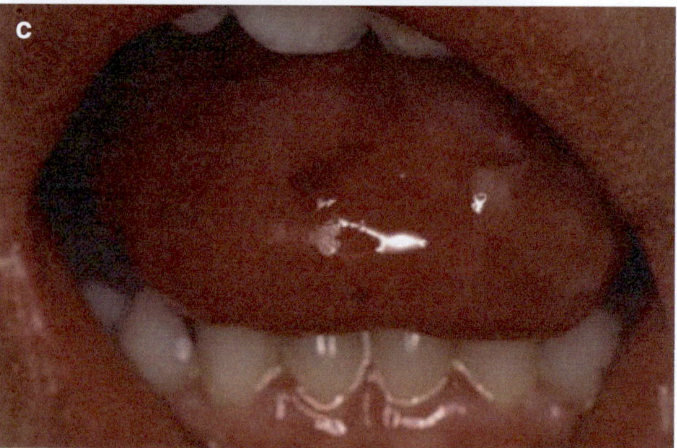

Summary

Severe illness in early childhood can have an adverse effect on enamel formation. Where genetic conditions feature enamel defects, they can either be directly attributable to gene expression patterns during amelogenesis or the result of the impact of systemic disease on ameloblast function. Very few conditions have been investigated in sufficient detail to precisely determine the pathogenesis of the enamel defect. In the future, modern in situ molecular technology should be able to demonstrate functional pathology of disease-causing gene products during odontogenesis, at least in an animal model of any given condition. Having said this, the mechanisms underpinning many dental anomalies remain mysterious even in some relatively common genetic or chromosomal anomalies such as trisomy 21, where anomalies of tooth number (hypodontia and hyperdontia) and microdontia are common. Although it may seem an obscure academic exercise to be aware of these rare conditions, there are occasions when accurate description of an enamel defect is an important step in diagnosing a rare disorder.

References

1. Jacobsen PE, Haubek D, et al. Developmental enamel defects in children born preterm: a systematic review. Eur J Oral Sci. 2014;122(1):7–14.
2. Arrow P. Risk factors in the occurrence of enamel defects of the first permanent molars among schoolchildren in Western Australia. Community Dent Oral Epidemiol. 2009;37(5):405–15.
3. Brogardh-Roth S, Matsson L, Klingberg G. Molar-incisor hypomineralization and oral hygiene in 10- to-12-yr-old Swedish children born preterm. Eur J Oral Sci. 2011;119:33–9.
4. Seow W. A study of the development of the permanent dentition in very low birthweight children. Pediatr Dent. 1996;18:379–84.
5. Oliver W, Owings C, Brown W, Shapiro B. Hypoplastic enamel associated with the nephrotic syndrome. Pediatrics. 1963;32:399–406.
6. Kagnoff M. Celiac disease: pathogenesis of a model immunogenetic disease. J Clin Invest. 2007;117(1):41–9.
7. Majorana A, Bardellini E, Ravelli A, Plebani A, Polimeni A, Campus G. Implications of gluten exposure period, CD clinical forms, and HLA typing in the association between celiac disease and dental enamel defects in children. A case-control study. Int J Paediatr Dent. 2010;20(2):119–24.
8. Aguirre J, Rodríguez R, Oribe D, Vitoria J. Dental enamel defects in celiac patients. Oral Surg Oral Med Oral Pathol Oral Radiol Endod. 1997;84:646–50.
9. Aine L. Coeliac-type permanent-tooth enamel defects. Ann Med. 1996;28(1):9–12.
10. Priovolou C, Vanderas A, Papagiannoulis L. A comparative study of enamel defects in children and adolescents with and without coeliac disease. Eur J Paediatr Dent. 2004;5(2):102–6.
11. Wierink C, Van Dierman D, Aartman I, Heymans H. Dental enamel defects in children with coeliac disease. Int J Paediatr Dent. 2007;17:163–8.
12. Maki M, Aine L, Lipsanen V, Koskimies S. Dental enamel defects in first-degree relatives of coeliac disease patients. Lancet. 1991;337:763–4.

13. Minicucci E, Lopes L, Crocci A. Dental abnormalities in children after chemotherapy treatment for acute lymphoid leukemia. Leuk Res. 2003;27(1):45–50.
14. Foster B, Nociti FH, Somerman MJ. The rachitic tooth. Endocr Rev. 2013;35:1–34. doi:10.1210/er.2013-1009.
15. Zambrano M, Nikitakis N, Sanchez-Quevedo M, Sauk J, Sedano H, Rivera H. Oral and dental manifestations of vitamin D-dependent rickets type I: report of a pediatric case. Oral Surg Oral Med Oral Pathol Oral Radiol Endod. 2003;95(6):705–9.
16. Hanna J, Niimi K, Chan J. X- linked hypophosphatemia: genetic and clinical correlates. Am J Dis Child. 1991;145(8):865–70.
17. Murayama T, Iwatsubo R, Akiyama S, Amano A, Morisaki I. Familial hypophosphatemic vitamin D-resistant rickets: dental findings and histologic study of teeth. Oral Surg Oral Med Oral Pathol Oral Radiol Endod. 2000;90(3):310–6.
18. Bender I, Naidorf I. Dental observations in vitamin D resistant rickets with special reference to periapical lesions. J Endod. 1985;11(11):514–20.
19. Alexander S, Moloney L, et al. Endodontic management of a patient with X-linked hypophosphataemic rickets. Aust Endod J. 2001;27(2):57–61.
20. Chaussain-Miller C, Sinding C, Septier D, Wolikow M, Goldberg M, Garabedian M. Dentin structure in familial hypophosphatemic rickets: benefits of vitamin D and phosphate treatment. Oral Dis. 2007;13(5):482–9.
21. Azevedo TDPL, Feijo GCS, Bezerra ACB. Presence of developmental defects of enamel in cystic fibrosis patients. J Dent Child. 2006;73(3):159–63.
22. Narang A, Maguire A, Nunn JH, Bush A. Oral health and related factors in cystic fibrosis and other chronic respiratory disorders. Arch Dis Child. 2003;88(8):702–7.
23. Sui W, Boyd C, Wright J. Altered pH regulation during enamel development in the cystic fibrosis mouse incisor. J Dent Res. 2003;82(5):388–92.
24. Flanagan N, O'Connor W, McCartan B, Miller S, McMenamin J, Watson R. Developmental enamel defects in tuberous sclerosis: a clinical genetic marker? J Med Genet. 1997;34(8):637–9.
25. OMIM. Online Mendelian Inheritance in Man. Center for Medical Genetics, Johns Hopkins University and National Center for Biotechnology Information. Baltimore: National Library of Medicine; 2013.
26. Balmer R, Fayle SAF. Enamel defects and ectopic eruption in a child with Usher syndrome and a cochlear implant. Int J Paediatr Dent. 2007;17(1):57–61.
27. Nordgarden H, Lima K, Skogedal N, Følling I, Storhaug K, Abrahamsen T. Dental developmental disturbances in 50 individuals with the 22q11.2 deletion syndrome; relation to medical conditions? Acta Odontol Scand. 2012;70(3):194–201.
28. Nieminen P, Lukinmaa P, Alapulli H, Methuen M, Suojärvi T, Kivirikko S, et al. DLX3 homeodomain mutations cause tricho-dento-osseous syndrome with novel phenotypes. Cells Tissues Organs. 2011;194(1):49–59.
29. Goodwin A, et al. Abnormal Ras signaling in Costello syndrome (CS) negatively regulates enamel formation. Hum Mol Genet. 2014;23(3):682–92.
30. Hunter L, Addy L, Knox J, Drage N. Is amelogenesis imperfecta an indication for renal examination? Int J Paediatr Dent. 2007;17(1):62–5.
31. Kantaputra P, Kaewgahya M, Khemaleelakul U, Dejkhamron P, Sutthimethakorn S, Thongboonkerd V, et al. Enamel-renal-gingival syndrome and FAM20A mutations. Am J Med Genet A. 2013;164A(1):1–9. Epub Nov 20.
32. Wright J. Oral manifestations in the epidermolysis bullosa spectrum. Dermatol Clin. 2010;28(1):159–64.
33. Luder H, Gerth-Kahlert C, Ostertag-Benzinger S, Schorderet D. Dental phenotype in Jalili syndrome due to a c.1312 dupC homozygous mutation in the CNNM4 gene. PLoS One. 2013;8(10):e78529.

Amelogenesis Imperfecta: Current Understanding of Genotype-Phenotype

5

John Timothy Wright

Abstract

There are nearly 100 hereditary conditions that affect enamel formation. Hereditary enamel conditions not associated with other tissue or developmental defects are traditionally referred to as amelogenesis imperfecta (AI). Enamel malformations involve either a deficiency in the amount of enamel (hypoplasia), a decrease in the mineral content or change in the composition of enamel (hypomineralization), or a combination of these two manifestations. The different amelogenesis imperfectas are challenging to diagnose and treat as they are extremely diverse in their clinical presentation and are genetically heterogeneous. There are multiple genes now known to cause AI and these different genes code for proteins that are critical for normal enamel formation. Ten genes with mutations known to cause AI have already been discovered, and the powerful new molecular technologies now available will help identify new genes that are associated with enamel defects. Understanding the etiology of hereditary conditions affecting enamel and how the enamel differs from normal (amount and/or composition) will allow clinicians to better advise their patients and select optimal treatment approaches.

Introduction

Enamel formation involves many diverse processes that are highly controlled at the molecular level. These processes and developmental pathways can be sensitive to environmental conditions that can disrupt the complex processes critical for normal biomineralization [1]. There are nearly 100 hereditary conditions that affect enamel formation that are recorded in the Online Mendelian Inheritance in Man

J.T. Wright, DDS, MS
Department of Pediatric Dentistry, University of North Carolina,
CB#7450 Brauer Hall, School of Dentistry, Chapel Hill, NC 27599-7450, USA
e-mail: tim_wright@dentistry.unc.edu

© Springer-Verlag Berlin Heidelberg 2015
B.K. Drummond, N. Kilpatrick (eds.), *Planning and Care for Children and Adolescents with Dental Enamel Defects: Etiology, Research and Contemporary Management*, DOI 10.1007/978-3-662-44800-7_5

database [2]. Most of these hereditary enamel defects are associated with syndromes where tissues other than enamel also are affected. Hereditary enamel conditions not associated with other tissue or developmental defects are traditionally referred to as amelogenesis imperfecta (AI) [3]. These hereditary conditions predominantly affect the quantity and/or quality of enamel in the absence of other developmental traits [4]. The different amelogenesis imperfectas are challenging to diagnose and treat as they are extremely diverse in their clinical presentation and are genetically heterogeneous. Prior to the identification of any genes known to cause AI, several studies described the prevalence and phenotype (clinical appearance) of AI [5–8] in a variety of populations around the world. Studies conducted in the United States, Israel [9, 10] and Scandinavian countries [9–13] indicate the prevalence of AI to range from about 1:700 to 1:14,000. It is likely that most general populations will have a prevalence of around 1:6,000–8,000 with the prevalence of specific subtypes varying in different populations. The purpose of this chapter is to provide clinicians with a guide that will help them identify the different AI types, the different causes of these conditions and how the specific genetic cause can be related to a specific clinical appearance or phenotype. How this knowledge is important for identifying a diagnosis and then for selecting different treatment approaches will also be addressed.

Classification of Amelogenesis Imperfecta

Since the first descriptions of hereditary enamel defects, a variety of nomenclatures and nosologies have been used for classifying the different AI types [14]. The various hereditary enamel defects were given descriptive names (e.g. hypoplastic, hypocalcified, yellow brown, etc.) depending on their clinical and histological features. Carl Witkop Jr. developed a classification system recognizing four main AI types that considered the phenotype, perceived pathogenesis and mode of inheritance: hypoplastic, hypomaturation, hypocalcified and hypomaturation-hypoplastic with taurodontism [4]. These main groups were then subdivided into 14 subtypes based on more distinctive clinical features and the Mendelian mode of inheritance. When this classification system was developed none of the genes causing these conditions were known, and it would indeed be nearly a quarter century before the first paper on an AI gene was published. Part of the Witkop classification was based on what he perceived was the underlying developmental mechanism or pathogenesis that would lead to the clinical phenotype [6]. Hypoplastic AI was considered a disturbance in ameloblasts where these enamel-forming cells did not generate enamel matrix adequately leading to a deficiency in amount or thickness of enamel. Hypomaturation AI was thought to be a defect in the specific stage of enamel development when proteinases were actively processing the remaining enamel matrix and final enamel crystallite growth occurred (maturation stage). The hypocalcified AI group was thought to be a defect in the biomineralization process of the enamel mineral that continued from initiation of mineralization through development of the entire enamel thickness. The enamel thickness in the hypomaturation and hypocalcified AI types was thought to be essentially normal as the ameloblasts were secreting the enamel matrix over the full thickness of the enamel, but the mineralization of the enamel was perturbed through these different mechanisms. Some AI cases were observed to have hypoplasia and hypomineralization of the enamel as well as taurodontism or apical displacement of the furcation in molar teeth [15]. Many of these cases were found to actually represent families with the tricho-dento-osseous syndrome [16].

As the molecular basis of the AI conditions have been elucidated and the phenotypes more carefully characterized using a variety of techniques, numerous investigators have called for a new nomenclature that includes the molecular basis of these conditions [17–19]. Indeed it became clear early on that there was a need to have a consistent nomenclature to describe the many different genetic mutations occurring in the same gene (allelic mutations) [20]. Standardized nomenclature has been adopted for classifying mutations for AI and other conditions and there have been some suggested changes in the AI classification but there is not at this time a classification system for AI that includes all the current genetic information [21]. Many clinicians still use the Witkop classification and it remains, for the most part, a useful way to communicate the phenotype and likely mode of inheritance. Several modifications to the Witkop classification have been proposed (Table 5.1) based on our increasing understanding of the pathogenesis of these conditions and these modifications attempt to simplify some of the subtypes that were based primarily on descriptive phenotypes (e.g., rough, smooth) [4, 22].

Inheritance of Amelogenesis Imperfecta

The early reports of enamel defects identified that they could be inherited by all the known modes of Mendelian inheritance: autosomal dominant, autosomal recessive and X-linked recessive [9]. The prevalence of the different subtypes varies with autosomal recessive AI types appearing to have a higher prevalence compared with the autosomal dominant AI types in Middle Eastern countries [10]. The presence of a family history of an enamel defect is very helpful in diagnosing whether the condition is indeed AI and what the AI subtype might be. Clinicians should ask patients and parents if anyone in the family has a similar enamel defect. If so, which family members and was there male-to-male transmission suggesting autosomal dominant inheritance. Were males and females similarly affected or did females often show a decreased level of severity? In the case of autosomal inherited traits, males and females will typically be similarly affected. However, if the trait is X-linked, males will typically have more severe manifestations compared with females due to lyonization [23]. Female cells only express one of their X chromosomes in any given cell so they will present a mosaic profile of affected and unaffected cells when they carry a mutation on a gene that resides on their X chromosome. Thus, enamel in females can be mildly or severely affected depending on the number of ameloblasts expressing DNA from the X chromosome with or without the mutant gene. This phenomenon of lyonization is clearly seen in the different X-linked AI subtypes where female enamel may be only mildly hypoplastic or variable in color changes that can present as streaks down the enamel of the tooth crown (Fig. 5.1) [24].

Table 5.1 Nomenclature and genetic basis for AI

Witkop classification	Modified classification	OMIM #	Gene
TYPE I hypoplastic			
IA – hypoplastic pitted (AD)	AD generalized hypoplastic	?	*LAMB3*
IB – hypoplastic local (AD)	AD generalized hypoplastic	104500	*ENAM*
IC – hypoplastic local (AR)	AR local hypoplastic	204650	*ENAM*
ID – hypoplastic smooth (AD)	AD generalized thin hypoplastic	?	?
IE – hypoplastic smooth (X linked)	X-linked generalized thin hypoplastic	301200	*AMELX*
IG – enamel agenesis (AR)	AR generalized thin hypoplastic (enamel-renal syndrome)	614253 204690	*FAM20A*
TYPE II hypomaturation			
IIA – pigmented hypomaturation (AR)	AR pigmented hypomaturation	(IIA1) 204700 (IIA2) 612529 (IIA3) 613211 (IIA4) 614832	*MMP20* *KLK4* *WDR72* *C4ORF*
IIB – hypomaturation (X linked)	X-linked hypomaturation	301200	*AMELX*
IIC – snowcapped (X linked)	X-linked snowcapped	301200	*AMELX*
TYPE III hypocalcified			
IIIA – hypocalcified (AD)	AD hypocalcified	130900	*FAM83H*
IIIB – hypocalcified (AR)	AR hypocalcified	Not listed	*SLC24A4*
TYPE IV hypomaturation-hypoplastic with taurodontism			
IVA – hypomaturation-hypoplastic with taurodontism (AD)	(AD) Tricho-dento-osseous syndrome	AI 104530 TDO 190320	*DLX3*
IVB – hypomaturation-hypoplastic with taurodontism (AR)	?	?	?

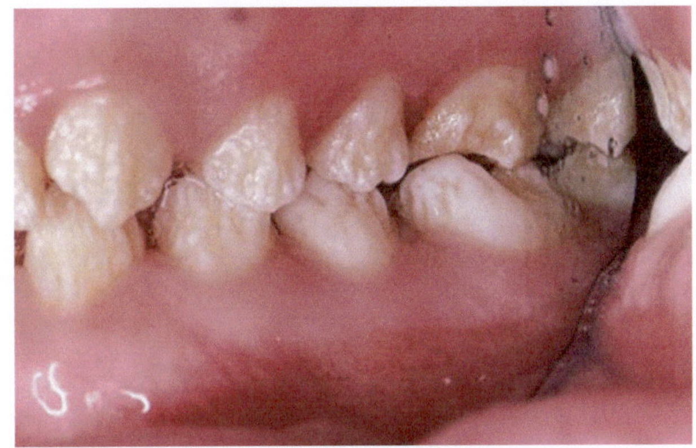

Fig. 5.1 All mutations in the *AMELX* gene that cause premature stop codons and loss of the C-terminus of the protein cause hypoplastic enamel. Females with these mutations will have variable areas of thick and thin enamel as seen in this affected female's permanent dentition

The clinical phenotypes seen with the different genetic mutations are markedly different. These phenotypic variations occur for several different reasons. There are multiple genes now known to cause AI and these different genes code for proteins that have diverse functions. Thus, it is not surprising that mutations in the amelogenin gene that codes for the most abundant enamel matrix protein (amelogenin) would be associated with a very different phenotype compared with mutations in a gene coding for a proteinase like MMP20 that is involved in processing the enamel matrix proteins. There are now over 10 different genes coding for different AI types as reviewed in Table 5.1 [19, 25–27]. These genes code for proteins that are part of the extracellular matrix, proteinases that process the matrix, proteins involved in cellular attachments, proteins involved in ion regulation, genes that regulate the expression of other genes and genes whose protein functions remain unknown at this time (Table 5.2).

Hypoplastic Amelogenesis Imperfecta

The primary feature of the different types of hypoplastic AI is some degree of thinning of the enamel. The currently known genes associated with this phenotype include *AMELX, ENAM, LAMB3,* and *FAM20A.* Currently all the *AMELX* mutations causing loss of protein due to signal peptide changes or loss of the C-terminus of the amelogenin protein result in a generalized thinning of the enamel layer in males and variable thinning in females (Fig. 5.1). Females with these types of *AMELX* mutations will have vertical furrows and grooves affecting the enamel thickness [20]. The difference in phenotype between males and females with X-linked AI is due to lyonization as described previously.

Many of the families identified as having autosomal recessive generalized hypoplastic amelogenesis imperfecta (OMIM #614253 AI and gingival fibromatosis syndrome) and mutations in the *FAM20A* gene have been shown to have microcalcifications in their kidneys and thus have enamel-renal syndrome (OMIM#204690) [28–30]. This condition has been reported using a variety of

Table 5.2 Amelogenesis imperfecta genes and function

Gene	Protein	Function[a]
AMELX	Amelogenin	Most abundant enamel matrix protein (90 %) important in enamel structure formation
ENAM	Enamelin	Enamel matrix protein important in crystallite elongation
WDR72	WD repeat domain 72	Intracellular protein may involve vesicle turnover
FAM83H	Family with sequence similarity 83, member H	Intracellular protein may involve keratin interaction
MMP20	Matrix metalproteinase 20	Removal of enamel matrix during secretory stage
KLK4	Kalikrien 4	Removal of enamel matrix during maturation stage
C4ORF26	Chromosome 4 open reading frame 26	Extracellular phosphoprotein with capacity to promote nucleation of mineral
DLX3	Distal-less 3 protein	Transcription factor
LAMB3	Laminin 5 beta chain	Cell attachment
SLC24A4	Solute carrier family 24 group4	Calcium transporter

[a]The specific function or functions of the different AI-associated genes and the proteins they produce are not well understood, and most of the purported protein functions listed remain to be confirmed and fully elucidated

names with the typical oral phenotype including generalized thin hypoplastic enamel, failure of eruption of teeth and gingival enlargement (Fig. 5.2a, b). Management of the dentition can be very difficult due to the combination of these features and the rather common occurrence of resorption of the unerupted teeth.

Mutations in the *ENAM* gene are associated with two distinct phenotypes. Mutations that cause a loss of protein are thought to result in a localized pitted phenotype due to haploinsufficiency (only a single functional copy of a gene) where a greatly diminished amount of protein is produced by the ameloblasts because only one of the two allelic *ENAM* genes produces a functional protein [31, 32]. This phenotype (OMIM#104500) is inherited as an autosomal dominant trait and is characterized by horizontal pitting or grooves that decorate the clinical crown. These hypoplastic pitted/grooved areas are juxtaposed between areas of enamel that are full thickness. The enamel color appears normal indicating a normal mineral content. Other *ENAM* mutations produce a generalized thin hypoplastic phenotype (OMIM#104500) through a dominant negative mechanism where it is thought that some dysfunctional protein is produced that interferes with the normal process causing a more global amelogenesis dysfunction and thin enamel over the entire dental crown. There are a few case reports of hypoplastic AI due to ENAM mutations being inherited through an autosomal recessive manner (OMIM#204650) [33].

Some presentations of AI have been shown to be associated with mutations that have effects in other tissues. Hypoplastic AI has recently been associated with mutations in genes that are important in cell-to-cell attachments such as *LAMB3* [27]. The protein product from the *LAMB3* gene and two other genes form the protein laminin 5 that is critical for anchoring the epidermis and dermis. Some

Fig. 5.2 (**a**) AR generalized thin hypoplastic AI with a failure of some teeth to erupt as seen in this 10-year-old females panoramic radiograph result from *FAM20A* mutations. (**b**) Clinically the teeth were small and spaced due to the very thin enamel, and the gingiva was fibrotic and overgrown in the maxillary anterior region. This affected individual also had multiple small calcifications in her kidneys consistent with the diagnosis of enamel-renal syndrome

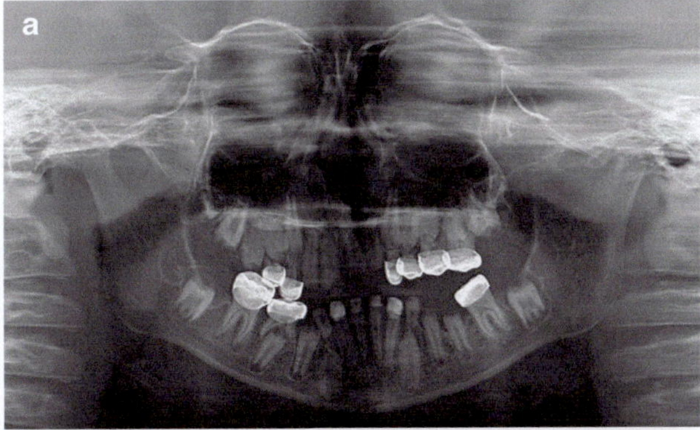

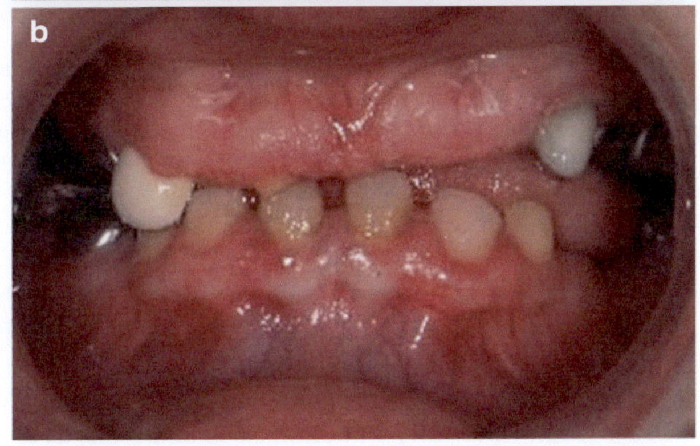

mutations in this gene are associated with junctional epidermolysis bullosa (OMIM# 226700, 226650) that is associated with tissue fragility and a propensity to develop large blisters and a hypoplastic pitted to generalized thin enamel phenotype [34]. Recently families with no predilection or history of blistering or skin manifestations have been identified to have *LAMB3* gene mutations associated with a hypoplastic enamel phenotype. It is likely that other genes important in cell-cell or cell-matrix interactions or other ameloblast critical functions will be found to be associated with hypoplastic enamel defects in the future. The majority of enamel defects reported with syndromes are of the hypoplastic phenotype although many of these conditions have not been fully characterized to determine if hypomineralization also is a phenotypic component.

Hypomaturation Amelogenesis Imperfecta

Hypomaturation AI phenotypes are associated with multiple genes that impact on the maturational process of amelogenesis (i.e. protein processing to allow crystallite mineralization and growth). Five genes are currently associated with this classification and phenotype (*AMELX, MMP20, KLK4, WDR72, C4ORF26*)

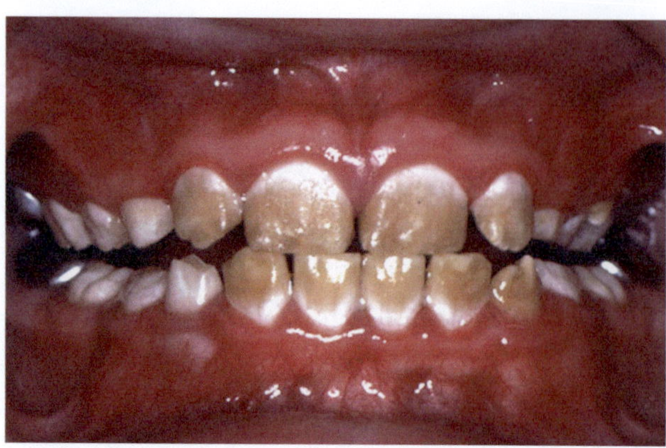

Fig. 5.3 The permanent dentition of males with the P70T mutation in the gene that codes for amelogenin have X-linked hypomaturation AI have a relatively normal enamel thickness with the coronol two thirds of the crown having a brown discoloration and the cervical area being white opaque in color. The primary molars all have a white opaque coloration

[19, 25, 35]. Mutations in the first three of these genes are known to involve processing of the enamel matrix. The role of WDR72 is not clear and the C4ORF26 protein may be important in regulation of crystallite mineralization. The clinical phenotype that results from all of these mutations includes enamel that is typically of normal thickness but is hypomineralized, has an increased protein content compared with normal fully mineralized enamel and as a result is abnormal in color and appearance [19]. Inheritance is either X-linked or autosomal recessive depending on the gene involved.

X-linked hypomaturation AI results from *AMELX* mutations that cause the amelogenin protein to be processed abnormally and at a slower rate [36]. For example, the *AMELX* P70T mutation causes a change of the proline amino acid at position 70 to a tyrosine and this alters a major proteinase cleavage site for MMP20, the primary proteinase for processing the amelogenin protein. In affected males, this results in enamel that in the primary dentition has a white opaque coloration and a brown coloration with a white opaque cervical enamel in the permanent dentition (Fig. 5.3) [37]. Females will have vertical striping of this discoloration due to lyonization [23].

The proteinases primarily responsible for processing the enamel matrix proteins (e.g. amelogenin, enamelin, ameloblastin, amelotin, etc.) are MMP20 and KLK4 [38]. Although MMP20 (a matrix metalloproteinase) is primarily active during the secretory stage of development, it is associated with hypomaturation AI due to its role in matrix processing that is a requisite for normal mineralization. KLK4 on the other hand is active in the maturation stage and is an aggressive serine proteinase that cleaves a variety of proteins to help ensure as much enamel matrix is processed and removed as possible to allow the enamel crystallites to grow and mineralize to the fullest extent. Enamel is normally about 85 % mineral per volume or 95 % by

Fig. 5.4 (**a**) All autosomal recessive hypomaturation AI types reported to date have a brown to orange coloration and enamel that is developmentally of normal thickness but that often fractures from the teeth as they erupt due to the enamel's reduced mineral content. (**b**) The panoramic radiograph of this female that has a WDR72 mutation shows the unerupted teeth have a normal outline of the crown, but there is little contrast between enamel and dentin due to their similar mineral content. The primary molars and maxillary incisors show marked enamel loss, while the first permanent molars also are beginning to show enamel fracturing

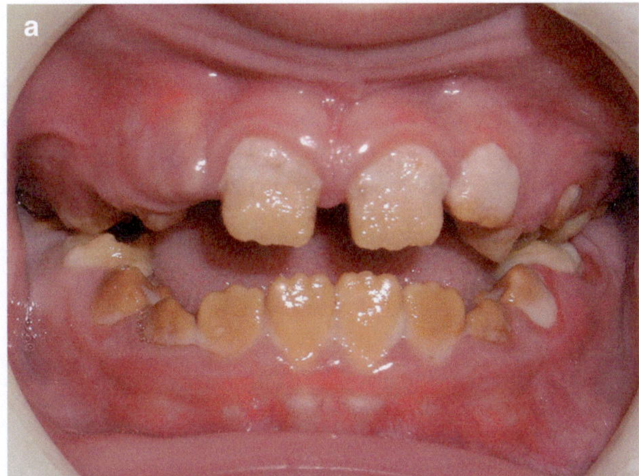
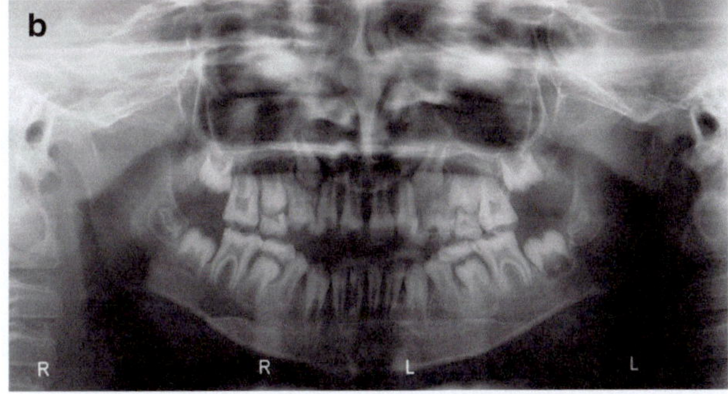

weight [39]. All of the hypomaturation AI types that have been characterized biochemically have retention of protein and decreased mineral content [40]. Interestingly, the mineral content varies substantially between the different hypomaturation AI types with the X-linked form having a higher mineral content than the proteinase-associated AI types, while the C4ORF26-associated AI has a very low mineral content and very high protein content [19, 24, 41]. Typically, the higher the protein content, the lower the mineral content and the more likely the affected individual is to have hypersensitivity of the teeth to thermal and chemical stimuli and loss of enamel as the teeth come into function.

The degree of enamel mineralization can be assessed clinically by features such as coloration of the dentition (discoloration is associated with decreased mineral content and increased protein content), enamel loss and fracturing and lack of radiographic contrast between enamel and dentin on radiographs (Fig. 5.4a, b). The presence and appearance of these phenotypic features can be helpful in determining which AI type an individual has as well as what the appropriate treatment might be. Enamel that is discolored, poorly mineralized, suffers fracturing from the crown and is associated with hypersensitivity displays phenotypic features that should lead the clinician to consider some type of full coronal coverage treatment.

Fig. 5.5 (**a**) Individuals with autosomal dominant hypocalcified AI typically have a markedly reduced mineral content and generalized yellow brown discoloration that affects all the teeth similarly as seen in the incisors of this child that has a FAM83H mutation. The teeth are frequently hypersensitive and it is common to have marked gingival irritation and heavy calculus formation. (**b**) Radiographically this 10-year-old child's enamel has been lost from all of the first permanent molars except around the cervical area. There is little contrast between enamel and dentin, and the unerupted crowns have a normal morphology

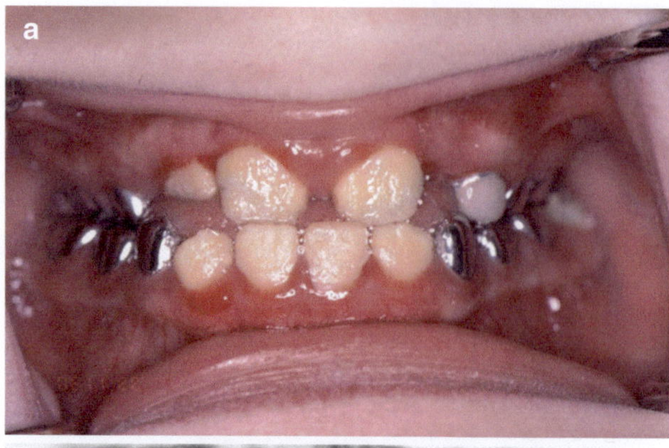

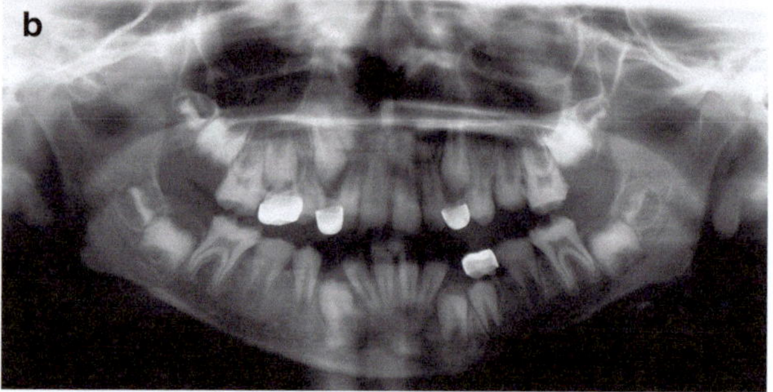

Hypocalcified Amelogenesis Imperfecta

The primary feature of hypocalcified AI is the marked reduction in the mineral content of the enamel that can be similar or even less than that of normal dentin. Most cases of hypocalcified AI are inherited as an autosomal dominant trait and are caused by mutations in the *FAM83H* gene. Typically all of the teeth in both the primary and permanent dentitions are similarly affected. The lack of mineral and increased protein content diminishes the insulating properties of the enamel and hypersensitivity is often a feature of this AI type. Affected individuals frequently have marked gingival inflammation and can have extensive calculus formation (Fig. 5.5a). The incompletely mineralized enamel contrasts poorly with the dentin on radiographs and tends to break away from the teeth as they come into function shortly after emergence into the oral cavity (Fig. 5.5b).

Some families have *FAM83H* mutations that are located farther in the 3-prime direction resulting in a genetic code that would generate a protein that is not as truncated as those produced by most FAM83H mutations. This slightly less truncated protein may have some functionality resulting in affected individuals having a localized hypocalcified phenotype with the cervical area of enamel typically being affected, while the rest of the dental crown is relatively normal. This is a relatively uncommon phenotype as most cases of hypocalcified AI involve the entire dental crown. There also can be autosomal recessive hypocalcified AI cause by mutations in the *SLC24A4* gene although these cases appear to be rare as well.

Hypomaturation/Hypoplastic Amelogenesis with Taurodontism

Taurodontism or elongation of the pulp chamber due to apical displacement of the floor of the pulp chamber and root furcation appears to occur with the different AI types with a prevalence similar to that in the general population [42]. Many of the cases reported in the literature as "AI with taurodontism" have later been recognized to be the autosomal dominant trait tricho-dento-osseous syndrome (TDO) that is caused by a mutation in the *DLX3* gene [42–44]. This gene regulates the expression of other genes and is involved in hair, tooth, and bone formation which are the three primarily affected tissues of the TDO syndrome. Two families with a different mutation in the *DLX3* gene do not display a bone phenotype and have a less severe, but noticeable, course hair phenotype [45, 46]. As increasing phenotypic variability is discovered from mutations in the same gene, it becomes evermore challenging to determine how best to classify and name these conditions.

Malocclusion and Amelogenesis Imperfecta

The presence of class III malocclusion with or without a skeletal open bite is much more prevalent in individuals with AI than the general population. Studies indicate around 25–45 % of individuals with AI will have these types of malocclusions [47, 48]. This phenotypic feature can occur in any of the AI types and is not always associated with self-reported dental hypersensitivity. It has been proposed that this could represent a direct effect of the mutated gene or may be a secondary effect. It seems likely that most of the open bite and class III malocclusions are not due directly to the dysfunctional mutant protein but due to other factors that remain unclear such as changes in bite force and tone of the muscles of mastication. These malocclusions certainly add greatly to the complexity, expense and duration of management of some AI cases.

Future Directions and Amelogenesis Imperfecta

The diagnosis of AI and its molecular causes at the gene level have advanced greatly since the first genetic mutation was identified in the amelogenin gene in 1991. New molecular techniques such as whole-genome sequencing make it possible to identify causative mutations with only a few affected individuals. Consequently, there are now 10 plus genes with mutations known to cause AI and there is no doubt that these powerful molecular technologies will help identify new genes that are associated with enamel defects. Knowing the molecular basis of the different AI types allows affected individuals and their families to have a definitive diagnosis that in the past was extremely challenging to obtain given the many types of AI and the diverse syndromic conditions that affect enamel formation. Clinicians that know the AI type and how the enamel is affected will be better able to identify treatment strategies and select the materials that are likely to generate optimal outcomes.

Understanding whether one should restore using bonding approaches or full-coverage restorations is often predicated on understanding how well or poorly the enamel is mineralized. It seems unlikely that there will be direct therapeutics related to our molecular understanding of the AI etiologies in the short term; however, this is occurring with other conditions and could be a possibility in the future.

References

1. Suckling G, Pearce E. Developmental defects of enamel in a group of New Zealand children: their prevalence and some associated etiological factors. Community Dent Oral Epidemiol. 1984;12:177–84.
2. OMIM, Online Mendelian Inheritance in Man. Center for Medical Genetics, Johns Hopkins University and National Center for Biotechnology Information, National Library of Medicine, Baltimore; 2013.
3. Weinmann J, Svoboda J, Woods R. Hereditary disturbances of enamel formation and calcification. J Am Dent Assoc. 1945;32:397.
4. Witkop CJJ. Amelogenesis imperfecta, dentinogenesis imperfecta and dentin dysplasia revisited, problems in classification. J Oral Pathol. 1989;17:547–53.
5. Rowley R, Hill FJ, Winter GB. An investigation of the association between anterior open-bite and amelogenesis imperfecta. Am J Orthod. 1982;81:229–35.
6. Witkop CJ, Sauk JJ. Heritable defects of enamel. In: Stewart, Prescott G, editors. Oral facial genetics. St. Louis: R. C.V. Mosby Company; 1976. p. 151–226.
7. Witkop C, Kuhlamnn W, Sauk J. Autosomal recessive pigmented hypomaturation amelogenesis imperfecta. Oral Surg Oral Med Oral Pathol. 1973;36(3):367–82.
8. Crawford P, Aldred M. Amelogenesis imperfecta: autosomal dominant hypomaturation-hypoplasia type with taurodontism. Br Dent J. 1988;164:71–3.
9. Witkop CJ. Hereditary defects in enamel and dentin. Acta Genet. 1957;7:236–9.
10. Chosack A, et al. Amelogenesis imperfecta among Israeli Jews and the description of a new type of local hypoplastic autosomal recessive amelogenesis imperfecta. Oral Surg. 1979;47:148–56.
11. Backman B. Amelogenesis imperfecta-clinical manifestations in 51 families in a northern Swedish country. Scand J Dent Res. 1988;96:505–16.
12. Backman B, Holm AK. Amelogenesis imperfecta: prevalence and incidence in a Northern Swedish County. Community Dent Oral Epidemiol. 1986;14:43–7.
13. Sundell S. Hereditary amelogenesis impertecta. An epidemiological, genetic and clinical study in a Swedish child population. Swed Dent J. 1986;31(Suppl):1–38.
14. Crawford PJ, Aldred M, Bloch-Zupan A. Amelogenesis imperfecta. Orphanet J Rare Dis. 2007;2:17.
15. Congleton J, Burkes E. Amelogenesis imperfecta with taurodontism. Oral Surg. 1979;48:540–4.
16. Wright JT, et al. Analysis of the tricho-dento-osseous syndrome genotype and phenotype. Am J Med Genet. 1997;72:197–204.
17. Aldred MJ, Crawford PJM. Amelogenesis imperfecta-towards a new classification. Oral Dis. 1995;1:2–5.
18. Wright JT, et al. Amelogenesis imperfecta: genotype-phenotype studies in 71 families. Cells Tissues Organs. 2011;194(2–4):279–83.
19. Parry DA, et al. Mutations in C4orf26, encoding a peptide with in vitro hydroxyapatite crystal nucleation and growth activity, cause amelogenesis imperfecta. Am J Hum Genet. 2012;91(3):565–71.
20. Wright JT, et al. Relationship of phenotype and genotype in X-linked amelogenesis imperfecta. Connect Tissue Res. 2003;44(suppl):72–8.

21. Hart PS, et al. Establishment of a nomenclature for X-linked amelogenesis imperfecta. Archs Oral Biol. 2002;47:255–60.
22. Nussier M, et al. Phenotypic diversity and revision of the nomenclature for autosomal recessive amelogenesis imperfecta. Oral Surg Oral Pathol Oral Med. 2004;97:220–30.
23. Witkop CJJ. Partial expression of sex-linked amelogenesis imperfecta in females compatible with the Lyon hypothesis. Oral Surgery Oral Med Oral Pathol. 1967;23:174–82.
24. Wright JT, et al. Enamel ultrastructure and protein content in X-linked amelogenesis imperfecta. Oral Surg Oral Med Oral Pathol. 1993;76(2):192–9.
25. Wright JT. The molecular etiologies and associated phenotypes of amelogenesis imperfecta. Am J Med Genet A. 2006;140(23):2547–55.
26. El-Sayed W, et al. Ultrastructural analyses of deciduous teeth affected by hypocalcified amelogenesis imperfecta from a family with a novel Y458X FAM83H nonsense mutation. Cells Tissues Organs. 2010;191(3):235–9.
27. Kim JW, et al. LAMB3 mutations causing autosomal-dominant amelogenesis imperfecta. J Dent Res. 2013;92(10):899–904.
28. Jaureguiberry G, et al. Nephrocalcinosis (enamel renal syndrome) caused by autosomal recessive FAM20A mutations. Nephron Physiol. 2012;122(1–2):1–6.
29. Wang SK, et al. FAM20A mutations associated with enamel renal syndrome. J Dent Res. 2014;93(1):42–8.
30. Kantaputra PN, et al. Enamel-renal-gingival syndrome and FAM20A mutations. Am J Med Genet A. 2014;164A(1):1–9.
31. Kim JW, et al. ENAM mutations in autosomal-dominant amelogenesis imperfecta. J Dent Res. 2005;84(3):278–82.
32. Hart PS, et al. Identification of the enamelin (g.8344delG) mutation in a new kindred and presentation of a standardized ENAM nomenclature. Archs Oral Biol. 2003;48: 589–96.
33. Hart TC, et al. Novel ENAM mutation responsible for autosomal recessive amelogenesis imperfecta and localized enamel defects. J Med Genet. 2003;40:900–6.
34. Wright JT, Hall KI, Grubb BR. Enamel mineral composition of normal and cystic fibrosis transgenic mice. Adv Dent Res. 1996;10:270–4.
35. El-Sayed W, et al. Mutations in the beta propeller WDR72 cause autosomal-recessive hypomaturation amelogenesis imperfecta. Am J Hum Genet. 2009;85(5):699–705.
36. Li W, et al. Reduced hydrolysis of amelogenin may result in X-linked amelogenesis imperfecta. Matrix Biol. 2001;19:7555–760.
37. Ravassipour DB, et al. Unique enamel phenotype associated with amelogenin gene (AMELX) codon 41 point mutation. J Dent Res. 2000;79:1476–81.
38. Simmer JP, Hu JC. Expression, structure, and function of enamel proteinases. Connect Tissue Res. 2002;43(2–3):441–9.
39. Robinson C, Weatherell JA, Hallsworth AS. Variations in the composition of dental enamel within thin ground sections. Caries Res. 1971;5:44–57.
40. Wright JT, Hall KI, Yamauchi M. The enamel proteins in human amelogenesis imperfecta. Archs Oral Biol. 1997;42:149–59.
41. Wright JT, et al. The mineral and protein content of enamel in amelogenesis imperfecta. Connect Tissue Res. 1995;31:247–52.
42. Seow WK. Taurodontism of the mandibular first permanent molar distinguishes between the tricho-dento-osseous (TDO) syndrome and amelogenesis imperfecta. Clin Genet. 1993;43:240–6.
43. Crawford PJM, Aldred MJ. Amelogenesis imperfecta with taurodontism and the tricho-dento-osseous syndrome: separate conditions or a spectrum of disease? Clin Genet. 1990;38:44–50.
44. Wright JT, et al. Phenotypic variability of the tricho-dento-osseous syndrome associated with a DLX3 homeobox gene mutation. In: Chemistry and biology of mineralized tissues. Proceedings of the sixth international conference. Goldberg M, Boskey A, Robinson C, editors. Amer Acad Orthoped Surg: Rosemont; 2000. p. 27–31.

45. Dong J, et al. DLX3 mutation associated with autosomal dominant amelogenesis imperfecta with taurodontism. Am J Med Genet A. 2005;133A(2):138–41.
46. Wright JT, et al. DLX3 c.561_562delCT mutation causes attenuated phenotype of tricho-dento-osseous syndrome. Am J Med Genet A. 2008;146(3):343–9.
47. Persson M, Sundell S. Facial morphology and open bite deformity in amelogenesis imperfecta. Acta Odontol Scand. 1982;40:135–44.
48. Cartwright AR, Kula K, Wright JT. Craniofacial features associated with amelogenesis imperfecta. J Craniofac Genet Dev Biol. 1999;19:148–56.

Molar Incisor Hypomineralization: Structure, Composition, and Properties

6

Erin K. Mahoney and Rami Farah

Abstract

The first permanent molars in molar incisor hypomineralization (MIH) are characterized by localized demarcated lesions or opacities within the enamel. These lesions are often rough and plaque retentive and at risk of rapid caries and post-eruptive breakdown (PEB). There is increasing evidence to suggest that the physical, chemical and mechanical properties of MIH-affected enamel are different to those of otherwise healthy enamel. Studies suggest that the hardness and modulus of elasticity of MIH-affected enamel are reduced by between 50 and 75 % and are accompanied by a simultaneous 20 % reduction in mineral content. Furthermore, the protein content of affected enamel is up to 15 times higher than in sound enamel particularly in the darker brown opacities. These findings may explain why hypomineralized enamel fractures easily under occlusal function causing PEB. Scanning and transmission electron microscopic studies have shown that the microstructure of this enamel is more disorganized and, when etched with phosphoric acid, it does not show the typical etching pattern. This may contribute clinically to the compromised bonding of adhesive dental materials to affected teeth. Knowledge of the physical and mechanical properties and composition of developmentally defective enamel helps clinicians understand the challenges associated with treating affected individuals.

E.K. Mahoney, BDS, MDSc PhD (✉)
Department of Dentistry, Hutt Valley District Health Board,
84 Te Anau Road, Hataitai, Wellington 6021, New Zealand
e-mail: Erin.Mahoney@huttvalleydhb.org.nz

R. Farah, BDS, MPhil, DClinDent, PhD
Department of Oral Sciences, University of Otago,
310 Great King Street, Dunedin 9016, New Zealand
e-mail: rami.farah@otago.ac.nz

© Springer-Verlag Berlin Heidelberg 2015
B.K. Drummond, N. Kilpatrick (eds.), *Planning and Care for Children and Adolescents with Dental Enamel Defects: Etiology, Research and Contemporary Management*, DOI 10.1007/978-3-662-44800-7_6

Introduction

The first permanent molars in children with MIH are characterized by localized demarcated hypomineralized enamel lesions or opacities with compromised mechanical properties. These hypomineralized lesions are often rough and plaque retentive which, coupled with hypersensitivity, makes adequate oral hygiene difficult. The net result is a predisposition to rapid caries and post-eruptive breakdown (Fig. 6.1). Over the past 15 years, there has been a growing body of research focused on understanding the physical and chemical properties and the behavior of such hypomineralized lesions. This is important as it helps clinicians to make informed treatment choices and provides greater insight into the likely long-term prognosis of these compromised teeth.

This chapter summarizes what is known about the structure, composition and properties of hypomineralized enamel and relates this knowledge to the clinical appearance and behavior of MIH-affected teeth. The first part of this chapter briefly reviews otherwise healthy sound enamel, while the second part describes the macro- and microscopic appearance of MIH enamel, its chemical and structural properties and their impact on its mechanical behavior.

Sound Enamel

Fully formed, sound enamel is 96 % weight and 86 % volume mineral (inorganic). It is produced by ameloblasts, which are highly specialized calcium transporting cells that are lost once amelogenesis is complete and the tooth erupts. Enamel is unique in the body, as it does not have the ability to heal or regenerate once tooth eruption is complete. The resulting enamel in health is a well-organized, highly mineralized, hard tissue that can withstand significant occlusal forces and the challenging oral environment.

Enamel mineral is initially a carbonated apatite which, through a process of maturation, is ultimately composed predominately of hydroxyapatite crystals ($Ca_{10}(PO_4)_6(OH)_2$) with trace elements such as magnesium, fluoride, strontium and lead. Although highly mineralized enamel does allow some movement of molecules,

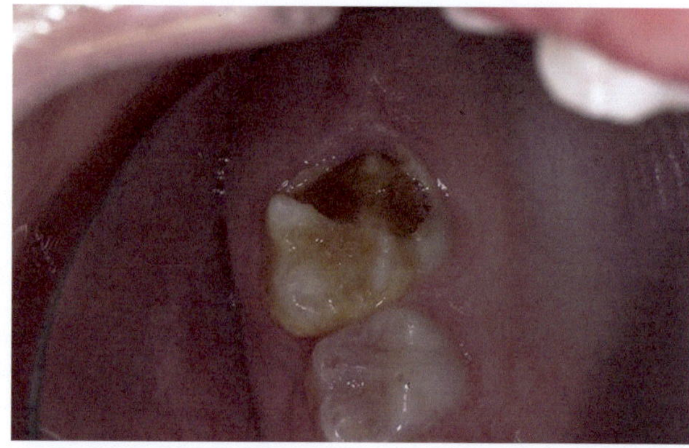

Fig. 6.1 An upper first permanent molar affected by MIH showing characteristic predisposition to post-eruptive breakdown superimposed with dental caries

in comparison to dentine its permeability in health is minimal. The orientation of the crystals together forms the rod structure (prism), which represents the "mineralized trail" taken by the ameloblasts and their Tomes processes as they migrate along an undulating course from the amelodentinal junction (ADJ) to the enamel surface. Enamel rods are between 3 and 7 μm in diameter. There are approximately 1,000 crystals found in each rod and each rod interdigitates with the neighboring ones. Where the rods meet, the crystals have different directions to this in the neighboring rods, thus creating a very narrow interface with slightly increased space between the crystals containing a greater abundance of organic matter. This area between the different rods is known as inter-rod areas or rod sheaths (Fig. 6.2).

Enamel does contain some organic material but only 1 % by weight (2 % by volume) and with a further 4 % water by weight (12 % by volume). The organic component of enamel is composed of proteins and lipids, which are produced mainly by the ameloblasts, although some may be derived from exogenous substances such as blood and serum. An area of higher concentration of organic material is found in the "tuft" region. Enamel tufts lie along with lamellae and spindles and are normal defects found in mature enamel but may represent an area of mechanical weakness. The role of the protein in enamel is still unclear but is thought to affect the behavior of this complex tissue, reducing its brittleness and imparting it with more metallic-like mechanical properties [1].

Hypomineralized Enamel

Macroscopic Changes

Clinically, MIH enamel defects appear as well-demarcated opacities within otherwise normal-looking enamel. These opacities are generally visible to the naked eye and vary in color from creamy-white to yellow or brown and affect the cuspal areas,

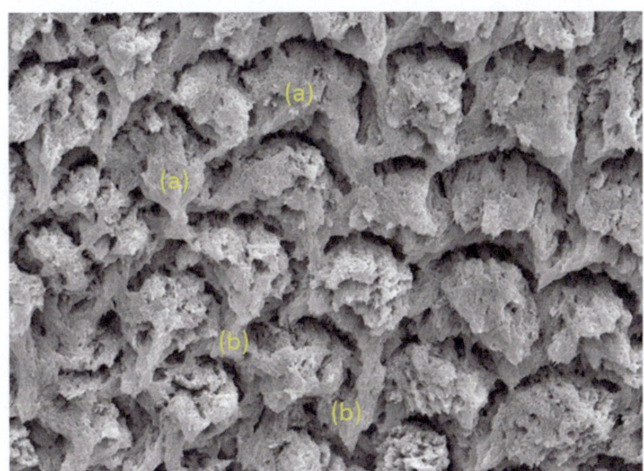

Fig. 6.2 Basic organization of the enamel rods as seen under the SEM. (**a**) Typical rod structure. (**b**) Inter-rod area (rod sheath)

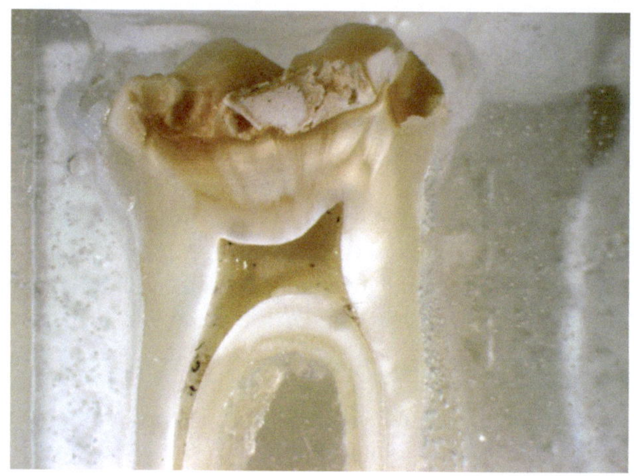

Fig. 6.3 A section through an extracted MIH-affected first permanent molar showing the lesion extending from the ADJ outwards through the occlusal surface with apparently unaffected cervical enamel

inclined planes and smooth surfaces. When MIH teeth, with clinically obvious opacities, are extracted and sectioned prior to any in vitro testing, the lesion usually extends from the ADJ to the surface of the tooth and the cervical enamel appears normal macroscopically (Fig. 6.3).

Mechanical Properties

The term "mechanical properties" refers to the characteristics of a material that determine how it reacts when subjected to some type of force. Understanding the mechanical properties of hypomineralized enamel helps clinicians predict the behavior of MIH-affected teeth. Two properties in particular, hardness and elastic modulus, have been the focus of most research. The hardness of a material provides a measure of its resistance to permanent indentation and is considered to reflect its susceptibility to abrasive wear. Elastic modulus provides information on how a material flexes under loading/pressure such as occlusal forces. Both hardness and elastic modulus testing rely on dropping an indenter of a known size and shape into the material under test. The size or depth of the resulting indent is measured, and the resulting "hardness" is calculated as pressure (force/area). The elastic modulus depends on the shape of the loading/unloading curve of the indenter and is also measured in the units of pressure. Unfortunately, different studies use different units such as GPa or Knoop hardness number (KHN), which makes inter-study comparisons difficult.

Sound enamel has a hardness of between 3.5 and 5.0 GPa while its modulus of elasticity is 77.25 ± 3.15 GPa (see Table 6.1) [2, 3]. This confirms that sound enamel is very hard and resistant to wear. In comparison sound dentine has a low wear resistance, with a hardness of around 0.83 GP and is more flexible than enamel with a modulus of elasticity of approximately 20–25 GPa [4]. Hypomineralized enamel has been shown to have mechanical properties that are similar to those of dentine as

Table 6.1 Hardness and modulus of elasticity of hypomineralized vs sound enamel

	Average hardness (GPa)	Average modulus of elasticity (GPa)
Sound enamel (control tooth)	3.66±0.75	75.57±9.98
Sound dentine	0.83±0.13	20–25
Hypomineralized enamel	0.53±0.31	14.49±7.56

opposed to those of sound enamel. Hardness values for enamel from hypomineralized first permanent molars have been reported as low as 0.5 GPa up to approximately 2 GPa with a modulus of elasticity of around 15 GPa [2, 3]. This 50–75 % reduction in the mechanical properties suggests that hypomineralized enamel has a low resistance to wear and will flex on loading which helps explain why MIH-affected teeth appear clinically weaker and more prone to fracture. Further work by Crombie and colleagues has shown that in general (although not always) white/cream-colored opacities are harder than yellow-brown lesions [2]. This information can be used clinically to help predict which teeth are likely to fracture or wear on eruption and which may be able to be monitored over time.

The mechanical properties of sound enamel do vary across the tooth surface [5–7]. This has also been found in the enamel of hypomineralized first permanent molars with the surface of the lesion being harder than the body [8]. Furthermore, there is a transitional zone between the apparently sound enamel of the cervical region and the hypomineralized defect (Fig. 6.4a–c). This transitional zone is approximately 500–600 μm (0.5–0.6 mm) in width, with a linear reduction in mechanical properties from the sound to affected enamel [9].

Studies have confirmed that the hardness and modulus of elasticity of enamel in the cervical region are essentially normal. This means that clinicians can expect this region to support normal bonding for restorative materials such as resin-based composites whereas adhesion in hypomineralized regions of enamel may be compromised.

Microstructure

In an attempt to explain why the mechanical properties of hypomineralized enamel differ so significantly from sound enamel, microstructural studies have been completed using both scanning electron microscopy (SEM) and transmission electron microscopy (TEM). SEM uses the reflection of a beam of electrons that are scanned across the surface of a specimen reflected to form an image. It allows detailed three-dimensional analysis of the surface of a given specimen. TEM allows for higher resolution by transmitting a beam of electrons through an ultrathin specimen. Depending on the composition and thickness of the specimen, some of the electrons are scattered and disappear and the unscattered electrons hit a fluorescent screen, which can be photographed or visualized directly. This allows investigation to a higher resolution than light microscopy and SEM.

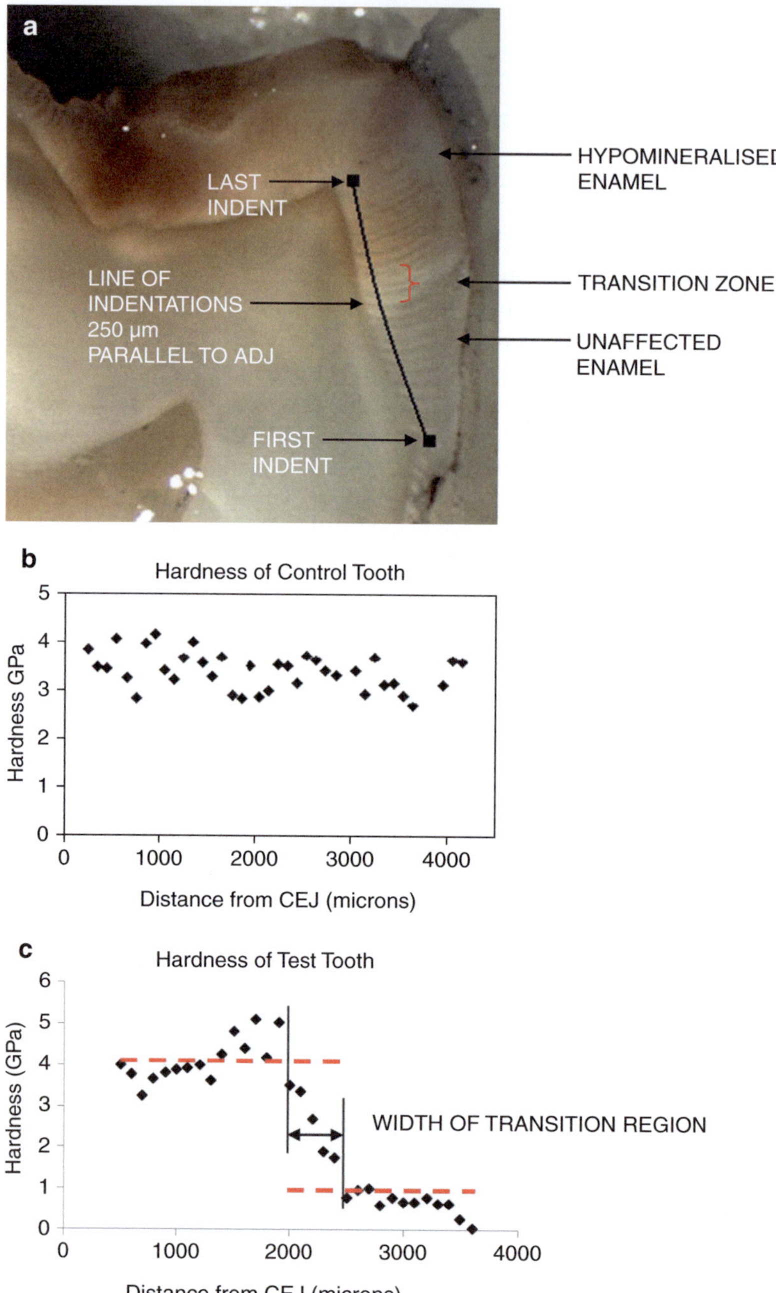

Fig. 6.4 (**a**) A cross section through an MIH-affected first permanent molar showing the transitional zone between the occlusal-affected enamel and the normal cervical enamel. (**b**) Hardness of unaffected control tooth from enamel at CEJ (cementoenamel junction) to a position level with the dentine cusp tip. (**c**) Hardness of first permanent molar seen in (**a**) showing the transitional area found between the sound and hypomineralized enamel

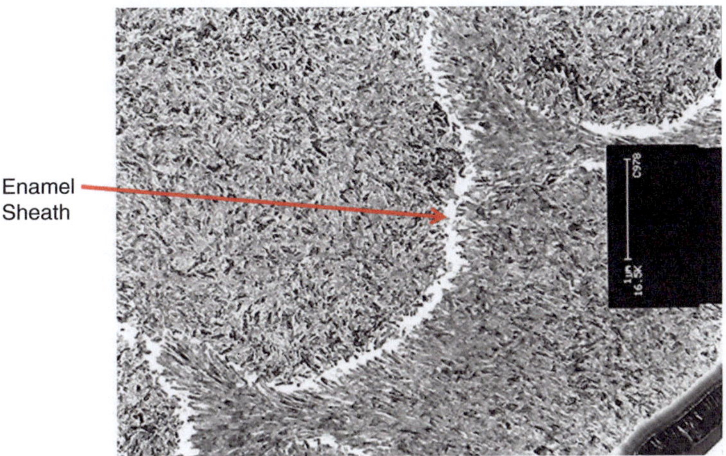

Fig. 6.5 A TEM image of hypomineralized enamel crystals showing the increased width of the enamel sheath structure (Courtesy of Zonghan Xie, Mark Hoffman, and Michael Swain)

The microstructure of sound enamel confirms its well-organized rod architecture and well-defined borders with narrow inter-rod regions without defects or porosities [10]. This also applies to the clinically normal looking, sound cervical enamel of MIH teeth. Under SEM, the affected enamel does show some of the basic architecture of the enamel rods, but there is always a varying degree of disorganization with increased porosities [9–11]. In moderately affected areas, the boundaries between the enamel rods are somewhat blurred, and the crystals are not tightly packed. In the more severely affected areas, the rods are very thin with wide gaps in between containing what appears to be organic material. The border between the normal cervical enamel and the affected occlusal part is always distinct. This can give clinicians further confidence when extending adhesive restorations onto the clinically normal-looking cervical enamel.

TEM studies of hypomineralized enamel are difficult to do as they require very thin samples for analysis. However, a few studies have been reported in which the higher magnification associated with TEM has allowed visualization of individual crystals within the enamel. TEM imaging of sound enamel shows that the apatite crystals are well organized with elongated crystals running along the long axis of the enamel rods. The rod sheaths are barely distinguishable and the organic material in this region is minimal. In contrast, TEM images of hypomineralized enamel have shown that this enamel is more porous and the crystals more loosely packed. The rod sheaths also show increased porosity making the sheath significantly wider than in sound enamel (see Fig. 6.5) [12]. It has been hypothesized that the wider sheath structure and less densely packed crystals mean that the enamel rods are more easily deformed under occlusal loading.

Restorative materials such as resin-based composites require micromechanical retention to bond effectively to the tooth surface. Successful adhesion to enamel is promoted by acid etching prior to placement of the resin-based material. The effect of phosphoric acid etchant on hypomineralized enamel is therefore important. SEM studies have consistently shown that, regardless of the etching time, exposure of hypomineralized enamel to phosphoric acid fails to produce any of the traditional etching patterns seen in sound enamel [13, 14]. It has been suggested that this abnormal etching pattern may be the result of excess proteins remaining in the compromised enamel preventing normal acid dissolution [10].

The microshear bond strength of a resin-based composite to hypomineralized enamel has been shown to be significantly less (up to a 54 % reduction) compared with that to sound enamel [13]. Furthermore, SEM studies confirmed a high frequency of cohesive failures within the compromised enamel as opposed to an adhesive failure at the interface with the composite material. This suggests that the hypomineralized enamel failed when stress was applied i.e. the enamel itself was weaker than the strength of the bond between the resin and compromised enamel.

The less densely packed crystals in the rods are associated with reduced mineral density and in turn compromised mechanical properties. Mineral density is an indication of the degree of mineralization of a given material. The higher the mineral density, the more mineralized the tissue and the more tightly packed the crystals. The reduced mineral density of MIH enamel has been confirmed using x-ray microtomography [15, 16]. This technique utilizes a small version of the computerized tomography (CT) scan to take multiple radiographic images of the specimen under study from multiple angles. A computer then uses the multiple radiographs to reconstruct a three-dimensional image of the specimen (in black and white as in conventional radiographs). Just as in conventional radiographs, the whiter the specimen (or enamel in this case), the more mineralized it is, and the darker the enamel, the less mineralized it is (hypomineralized). This is referred to as the gray-level reading of the enamel. The gray level can be read (given a number) depending on how white or dark it is, and this number can then be used to directly calculate the mineral density of enamel. The mineral density of affected MIH enamel is, on average, around 20 % lower than that of sound enamel and varies across the lesion [15]. Cervically, where the enamel appears clinically normal, the mineral density is normal; however it drops across the transitional zone into the affected occlusal region. The mineral density is lowest in the center of the lesion. Using x-ray microtomography it was also demonstrated that the MIH defects follow the incremental lines of enamel formation. Three dimensionally, this suggests that defects are shaped like an irregular cone, with the narrow tip located close to the ADJ and the wider base fanning out towards the enamel surface.

In addition to a reduction in the mineral density, the less densely packed crystals are associated with a 5–25 % increase in porosity as demonstrated using polarized light microscopy [2, 11, 17]. The high porosity in MIH enamel, combined with wide dentinal tubules, may allow for easier irritation of the thermal and chemical stimuli to the pulp. Rodd and co-workers demonstrated quantitative changes in the pulpal tissue of hypomineralized teeth, with increased neuronal and vascular expression of a noxious heat receptor in some pulpal regions [18]. This is indicative of underlying pulpal inflammation. Clinically, this inflammation leads to heightened pulpal excitability and sensitivity in the affected teeth, making a simple procedure like brushing the teeth or drinking a cold or a warm beverage difficult for MIH-affected individuals. This hypersensitivity can also make it difficult to achieve adequate local anesthesia. The use of local anesthesia supplemented by sedation or systemic pain relief can be helpful in treating affected children [19, 20].

There is a link between the color or shade of the enamel and the severity of the defect. Clinically, the darker the enamel i.e. yellow-brown as opposed to white-chalky, the more porous it is and the less its mineral density [17, 21]. This suggests that the darker the enamel opacity, the more likely it is to fracture under normal occlusal loads which has been demonstrated in one prospective cohort study [22].

Composition

Enamel is made up of two phases: an inorganic (mineral) phase of hydroxyapatite crystals and an organic phase of mainly proteins and some lipids. The proteins are mainly intrinsic enamel proteins such as enamelin and amelogenin.

The inorganic component of MIH enamel has been studied extensively using a variety of methods. The conventional calcium hydroxyapatite crystals found in normal enamel is the only calcium phosphate phase present in MIH enamel [3]. The calcium and phosphate content is lower in MIH enamel than in sound enamel [23], but they have similar Ca/P ratios. However, MIH-affected enamel has increased carbon content which reflects an increase in both carbonate [2] and protein content [24]. The increase in carbonate makes the affected enamel more susceptible to dental caries because carbonated crystals dissolve more easily under caries acid attack. However, the increased protein content increases enamel resistance to acid attack, as the proteins are more resistant to acid dissolution. As a result the association between caries and MIH remains unclear.

As for other trace elements, there is probably a slightly higher amount of magnesium in MIH enamel than in sound enamel, which suggests some form of disruption to amelogenesis. However, concentrations of chlorine, strontium, sodium, and potassium in MIH enamel are comparable (or slightly higher) to those in sound enamel [9, 23].

As mentioned earlier there is an inverse relationship between the clinical appearance of the opacities seen in MIH and its mineral density, with darker lesions containing less mineral. Conversely, there is a positive correlation between the shade and the amount of protein contained in these lesions. Studies have shown that brown MIH enamel has a 15–21-fold higher protein content than sound enamel. The protein content of both white/opaque and yellow enamel is approximately eight times higher than sound enamel [21, 24]. Increases in protein content have also been reported in the hypomineralized enamel that characterizes both hypomaturation and hypocalcified amelogenesis imperfecta (AI) types (see Chap. 5) [25, 26]. However, while the proteins identified in AI enamel are mainly intrinsic enamel proteins (e.g., amelogenins, enamelins), those found in MIH enamel are mainly serum and blood proteins. Indeed MIH enamel has been reported to have essentially normal levels of amelogenins [27]. The main protein found in MIH enamel is albumin with other serum proteins, such as alpha-1-antitrypsin and antithrombin III also present.

Hemoglobin and proteins involved in tissue injury and its repair, or in bleeding and coagulation, have also been detected, but with less abundance than serum proteins [24, 27].

The presence of serum proteins in MIH enamel is peculiar. While minute amounts of albumin and other serum proteins do enter enamel during development, they are degraded and removed during the maturation phase [28]. Only trace amounts are detected in mature sound enamel. It is unclear how such an abundance of serum proteins (and some hemoglobin) can gain access into MIH enamel. The most likely explanation is that there is "leakage" of serum (and perhaps blood) into MIH enamel during its formation. If this leakage occurs during the transition and maturation stages of amelogenesis it is likely to have a detrimental effect because albumin has the capacity to bind to the immature apatite crystals, inhibiting their growth [29]. In normal enamel formation, albumin degradation in the maturation stage is a prerequisite for maximal crystal growth. In addition, alpha-1-antitrypsin and antithrombin are serine proteinase inhibitors, interfering with the function of the proteinase kallikrein 4 (KLK4). KLK4 secreted during these stages of amelogenesis degrades the organic matrix remaining from the secretion stage. This facilitates the continued deposition of minerals into enamel required for full mineralization of hard enamel. The presence of antitrypsin and antithrombin may impair KLK4 activity resulting in hypomineralized enamel with the associated elevated protein and reduced mineral content.

Conclusion

The structure, composition, and properties of hypomineralized enamel are fundamentally altered which in turn affects its behavior and response to both the oral environment and dental treatment. Biomaterial science and scientists, through the use of a variety of in vitro techniques, can help clinicians understand these differences. Further research, which should also extend to hypomineralized primary enamel, is required to identify ways to optimize mineralization of developmentally defective enamel and to improve both prevention and treatment strategies in the future.

References

1. He LH, Swain MV. Enamel – a "metallic-like" deformable biocomposite. J Dent. 2007; 35(5):431–7.
2. Crombie FA, Manton DJ, Palamara JE, Zalizniak I, Cochrane NJ, Reynolds EC. Characterisation of developmentally hypomineralised human enamel. J Dent. 2013;41(7):611–8.
3. Mahoney E, Ismail FS, Kilpatrick N, Swain M. Mechanical properties across hypomineralized/hypoplastic enamel of first permanent molar teeth. Eur J Oral Sci. 2004;112(6): 497–502.
4. Kinney JH, Marshall SJ, Marshall GW. The mechanical properties of human dentin: a critical review and re-evaluation of the dental literature. Crit Rev Oral Biol Med. 2003;14(1):13–29.

5. Cuy JL, Mann AB, Livi KJ, Teaford MF, Weihs TP. Nanoindentation mapping of the mechanical properties of human molar tooth enamel. Arch Oral Biol. 2002;47:281–91.
6. Meredith N, Sherriff M, Setchell DJ, Swanson SAV. Measurement of the mircohardness and Young's modulus of human enamel and dentine using an indentation technique. Arch Oral Biol. 1996;41:539–45.
7. Xu HHK, Smith DT, Jahanmir S, Romberg E, Kelly JR, Thompson VP, et al. Indentation damage and mechanical properties of human enamel and dentin. J Dent Res. 1998;77(3):472–80.
8. Crombie F, Cochrane NJ, Manton DJ, Palamara JE, Reynolds EC. Mineralisation of developmentally hypomineralised human enamel in vitro. Caries Res. 2013;47:259–63.
9. Mahoney EK, Rohanizadeh R, Ismail FS, Kilpatrick NM, Swain MV. Mechanical properties and microstructure of hypomineralised enamel of permanent teeth. Biomaterials. 2004;25(20):5091–100.
10. Jalevik B, Dietz W, Noren JG. Scanning electron micrograph analysis of hypomineralized enamel in permanent first molars. Int J Paediatr Dent. 2005;15(4):233–40.
11. Suckling GW, Nelson DG, Patel MJ. Macroscopic and scanning electron microscopic appearance and hardness values of developmental defects in human permanent tooth enamel. Adv Dent Res. 1989;3(2):219–33.
12. Xie Z, Kilpatrick NM, Swain MV, Munroe PR, Hoffman M. Transmission electron microscope characterisation of molar-incisor-hypomineralisation. J Mater Sci Mater Med. 2008;19(10):3187–92.
13. William V, Burrow MF, Palamara JEA, Messer LB. Microshear bond strength of resin composite to teeth affected by molar hypomineralization using 2 adhesive systems. Pediatr Dent. 2006;28(3):233–41.
14. Mahoney EK. Micromechanical and structural analysis of compromised dental tissues. PhD thesis, University of Sydney; 2005.
15. Farah RA, Swain MV, Drummond BK, Cook R, Atieh M. Mineral density of hypomineralised enamel. J Dent. 2010;38(1):50–8.
16. Fearne J, Anderson P, Davis GR. 3D X-ray microscopic study of the extent of variations in enamel density in first permanent molars with idiopathic enamel hypomineralisation. Br Dent J. 2004;196(10):634–8. Discussion 25.
17. Jalevik B, Noren JG. Enamel hypomineralization of permanent first molars: a morphological study and survey of possible aetiological factors. Int J Paediatr Dent. 2000;10(4):278–89.
18. Rodd HD, Boissonade FM, Day PF. Pulpal status of hypomineralized permanent molars. Pediatr Dent. 2007;29(6):514–20.
19. Kilpatrick NM. New developments in understanding development defects of enamel: optimizing clinical outcomes. J Orthod. 2009;36:277–82.
20. Jalevik B, Klingberg GA. Dental treatment, dental fear and behaviour management problems in children with severe enamel hypomineralization of their permanent first molars. Int J Paediatr Dent. 2002;12(1):24–32.
21. Farah RA, Drummond BK, Swain M, Williams S. Linking the clinical presentation of molar-incisor hypomineralisation to its mineral density. Int J Paediatr Dent. 2010;5:353–60.
22. Da Costa-Silva CM, Ambrosano GMB, Jeremias F, De Souza JF, Mialhe FL. Increase in severity of molar–incisor hypomineralization and its relationship with the colour of enamel opacity: a prospective cohort study. Int J Paediatr Dent. 2011;21(5):333–41.
23. Jalevik B, Odelius H, Dietz W, Noren J. Secondary ion mass spectrometry and X-ray microanalysis of hypomineralized enamel in human permanent first molars. Arch Oral Biol. 2001;46(3):239–47.
24. Farah RA, Monk BC, Swain M, Drummond BK. Protein content of molar-incisor hypomineralisation enamel. J Dent. 2010;38(7):591–6.
25. Parry David A, Brookes Steven J, Logan Clare V, Poulter James A, El-Sayed W, Al-Bahlani S, et al. Mutations in C4orf26, encoding a peptide with in vitro hydroxyapatite crystal nucleation and growth activity, cause amelogenesis imperfecta. Am J Hum Genet. 2012;91(3):565–71.

26. Wright JT, Hall KI, Yamauchi M. The enamel proteins in human amelogenesis imperfecta. Arch Oral Biol. 1997;42(2):149–59.
27. Mangum JE, Crombie F, Kilpatrick NM, Manton DJ, Hubbard MJ. Surface integrity governs the proteome of hypomineralised enamel. J Dent Res. 2010;69:1160–5.
28. Robinson C, Brookes SJ, Kirkham J, Shore RC, Bonass WA. Uptake and metabolism of albumin by rodent incisor enamel in vivo and postmortem: implications for control of mineralization by albumin. Calcif Tissue Int. 1994;55(6):467–72.
29. Robinson C, Kirkham J, Brookes SJ, Shore RC. The role of albumin in developing rodent dental enamel: a possible explanation for white spot hypoplasia. J Dent Res. 1992;71(6): 1270–4.

The Psychosocial Impacts of Developmental Enamel Defects in Children and Young People

Zoe Marshman and Helen D. Rodd

Abstract

Within pediatric healthcare, increasing importance is being placed on the patient's own experience of illness and related treatments. Clearly there is a need for dentists to also appreciate how various oral conditions may impact on their young patients. The dental literature has a long tradition of epidemiological, clinical, and laboratory research relating to developmental defects of enamel (DDE). Psychosocial research, however, is a more recent line of enquiry, and one that is still in its infancy, particularly where children and young people are concerned. In this chapter we will consider how disturbances in enamel formation can affect the appearance and function of teeth which, in turn, can impact on an individual's emotions and social interactions. In addition, the need for patients to undergo, sometimes complex and prolonged, courses of treatment may bring its own positive or negative effects. We will first broadly consider the various approaches that can be used to gain insight into children's perspectives of oral conditions and dental treatment. The psychosocial impacts of DDE will then be described in terms of how they affect the individual, how dental interventions affect the individual, and, lastly, how others view young people with DDE.

Z. Marshman, BDS, MPH, DDPH, PhD (✉)
Academic Unit of Dental Public Health, School of Clinical Dentistry, University of Sheffield, Claremont Crescent, Sheffield, South Yorkshire S10 2TA, UK
e-mail: z.marshman@sheffield.ac.uk

H.D. Rodd, BDS (Hons), PhD
Department of Oral Health and Development, School of Clinical Dentistry, University of Sheffield, Claremont Crescent, Sheffield, South Yorkshire S10 2TA, UK
e-mail: h.d.rodd@sheffield.ac.uk

© Springer-Verlag Berlin Heidelberg 2015
B.K. Drummond, N. Kilpatrick (eds.), *Planning and Care for Children and Adolescents with Dental Enamel Defects: Etiology, Research and Contemporary Management*, DOI 10.1007/978-3-662-44800-7_7

Introduction

Over the last decade, there has been growing appreciation of the relationship between oral health status and children's quality of life or well-being. This has led to a wealth of studies exploring the impact of dental disease, dentoalveolar trauma, malocclusion, and dental or craniofacial anomalies on both oral health-related and general health-related quality of life [1–6]. Furthermore, greater emphasis is now being placed on young patients' perspectives and experiences of dental care and their participation in decision-making [7]. It is speculated that changes in how children are viewed and engaged in dentistry may underpin and facilitate future enamel defect-related research and service evaluation.

Research into the impacts of DDE may be driven by different agendas. Firstly, at the population level, there has been a need to establish whether DDE constitute a public health concern in the ongoing debate about the risks/benefits of water fluoridation. Indeed, the majority of psychosocial DDE-related research to date has been conducted in areas of natural or artificial water fluoridation in both developed and developing countries. Secondly, at the patient level, clinicians need to fully understand the impacts of DDE for each individual in order to better meet their needs and treatment expectations.

The media and celebrity industry also play a key role in shaping how society views and values appearance. Many children are growing up in a world where unrealistic body images are portrayed as desirable. A "perfect" smile of straight and artificially white teeth is inherent to this globalized representation of beauty. There is little tolerance for tooth color that deviates from the norm, placing a greater psychosocial impact on the individual and presenting more complex clinical and ethical challenges for the dentist.

Child-Centered Approaches to Research and Service Evaluation

A variety of methods, both qualitative and quantitative, may be used to engage children in research about their oral health and experiences of treatment [8]. Oral health-related quality of life (OHRQoL) questionnaires have dominated quantitative research in this field. The most frequently used child measures include the age-specific Child Perceptions Questionnaires (CPQ_{11-14} and CPQ_{8-10}) [9–11], the Child Oral Health Impact Profile (Child OHIP) [12], and the Child Oral Impacts on Daily Performances (Child OIDP) Questionnaire [13]. It should be borne in mind that these instruments are generic OHRQoL measures, and although they have been used with children with DDE [1, 14–16], they are not specific for enamel conditions. Studies have also employed proxy (parent) assessments of child OHRQoL in relation to DDE [2], but these will not be reviewed in this chapter as the focus is on children's self-reported impacts. Multidisciplinary research has also examined the relationship between the impact of DDE and various psychological constructs such as coping styles or self-esteem [17, 18].

In view of the recognized limitations of questionnaires in capturing the full spectrum of an individual's experiences, qualitative methods have been used to gain a more detailed insight into the impacts of DDE. Common approaches have included interviews, focus groups, and written diaries [16, 19–22], but there is considerable scope to utilize more diverse participatory activities such as video diaries, photo-elicitation, creative writing, drawings, and role play.

Psychosocial Impacts of Enamel Defects on the Individual

Background

As mentioned previously, both qualitative and quantitative approaches have been employed to determine the impacts of DDE on children, with greatest insights gained from studies which have incorporated a mixed method approach. A key finding to emerge from the literature is that there is no clear relationship between the severity of the condition, as measured by normative data (e.g., epidemiological indices of enamel defects), and the impact of DDE from the child's own perspective [23, 24]. This may be attributed to the complex interplay between individual characteristics such as coping strategies and concepts of the self (e.g., self-esteem and self-confidence) which may all modify a person's response to having a visible difference [20, 24–26]. One area which remains completely un-researched is whether the etiology of the DDE, inherited or environmental, has any bearing on the reported impacts. The prevalence of DDE in the general population has, however, been considered as a modifying factor on how children feel about their teeth. Interestingly, there are conflicting reports as to whether children living in areas where DDE are the "norm" (regions of endemic dental fluorosis) actually experience any less negative impacts relating to social interactions and satisfaction with their appearance [27–29]. The following sections will review some of the key studies which have described or measured impacts in young populations relating to a variety of DDE.

Impacts Relating to Dental Fluorosis

In the main, the psychosocial literature has focussed on children with DDE on permanent teeth attributed to dental fluorosis [28] and less is known about how conditions such as amelogenesis imperfecta (AI), molar incisor hypomineralization (MIH), or trauma-related sequelae affect individuals.

One of the earliest studies to consider the psychosocial impact of severe dental fluorosis was conducted with 13- to 15-year-olds living in Tanzania [27]. The main finding was that 70 % of respondents said that the way their teeth looked hindered them from smiling freely. Interestingly, the negative impact of DDE on smiling has been a common theme throughout the literature.

A more detailed investigation was later carried out in Tanzania, in an area where 75 % of the population had a Thylstrup-Fejerskov Index (TFI) score of ≥ 2 [14]. To

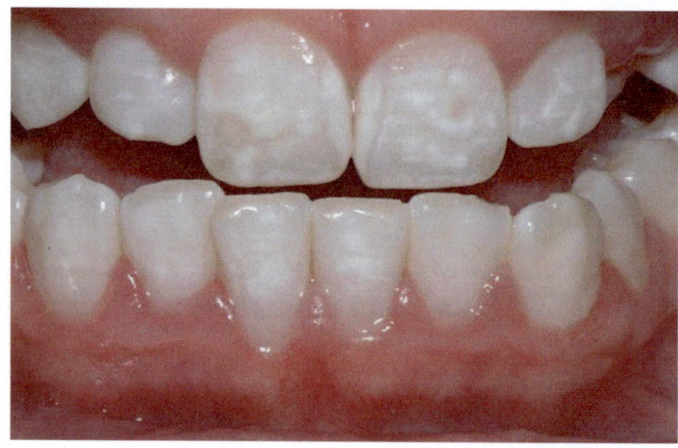

Fig. 7.1 Photograph of teeth of a participant with development enamel defects who said: "I always wanted to change my teeth, they are like multi-coloured… I'm loads bothered" (girl, aged 14)

appreciate the appearance of teeth which may be classified as having a TFI of 4 or 9, see Figs. 7.1 and 7.4, respectively. A sample of 478 young people, with a mean age of 15.7 years, completed a modified version of OIDP. They were asked how often they had experienced problems with their mouth or teeth in relation to seven daily performances: eating, speaking and pronouncing clearly, cleaning teeth, sleeping and relaxing, smiling without embarrassment, maintaining emotional state, and enjoying contact with people. Significantly more females than males reported themselves to be affected on at least one daily performance. Overall, young people who reported either oral impacts on their daily performance and/or discoloration of upper anterior teeth were more likely to be dissatisfied with both their oral condition and their dental appearance.

A similar study in Brazil also investigated the impact of fluorosis using a modified version of OIDP, this time with 513 schoolchildren aged 6–15 years [15]. No differences in impact on daily activities (eating, speech, oral hygiene, sleep, smiling, emotional stability, studying, and socializing) were found between those normatively assessed as having fluorosis or not. Robinson and coworkers [30] issued the CPQ_{11-14} to a sample of 174 12-year-old Ugandan children, 24 % of whom had dental fluorosis. They reported that more participants with socially noticeable fluorosis (TFI>2) had impacts on their OHRQoL than those with mild or no fluorosis, although the difference was not significant.

Studies in developed countries, where any fluorosis is likely to be less severe, have suggested that there is no impact on OHRQoL [1, 31]. Indeed, a study of 8- to 13-year-old Australian children found that those with a TFI of 2 had better OHRQoL than their peers with normal enamel [1]. However, it was not clear whether this could be attributed to the "whiteness" of affected teeth or reduced caries incidence.

Impacts Relating to Amelogenesis Imperfecta

Although there have been comparatively few studies on the psychosocial aspects of AI [32], it is evident that this condition has far greater impact than dental fluorosis. This is not surprising in view of the often severe functional problems, relating to dental hypersensitivity and tooth tissue loss, which may accompany compromised aesthetics. The first, and landmark, study of the psychosocial impacts of AI was conducted with a mainly adult population, although a few adolescent participants were included [19]. Interestingly, social avoidance and distress were found to be greatest among younger patients. More recently, a mixed method study involving children from a UK dental hospital has made a significant contribution to our understanding of how AI affects younger people [16]. In-depth interviews were conducted with seven children, aged 13–16 years. A further 40 AI patients, aged 10–16 years, completed the CPQ_{11-14} as well as some additional questions generated from the previous interviews. Participants reported impacts relating to aesthetics as well as function. Children did not like to show their teeth, especially for photographs and in social settings.

> I don't like smiling with my teeth because I don't like them (girl, aged 13)

> When all my friends are talking I'd want to join in but don't want to show my teeth (girl, aged 16)

For some children, tooth sensitivity was actually more of an issue than aesthetics.

> It is the sensitivity more than the colour, the colour doesn't bother me, it's more the sensitivity (girl, aged 15)

> If there was no problem with sensitivity, I'd drink faster and bite down on ice lollies and not cringe when I think of it (girl, aged 13)

Impacts Relating to DDE of Unknown Etiology

The only study to utilize in-depth interviews to explore the impact of DDE was conducted in the UK with populations receiving either a non-fluoridated or fluoridated (1 ppm) water supply [23]. A theoretical framework, based on symbolic interactionism was used to guide and interpret the qualitative data. Twenty-one 10- to 15-year-old young people were interviewed, with TFI scores ranging from 0 to 5. The impact of DDE was frequently described in terms of how much dental appearance "bothered" the individual. Photographs of the teeth of two participants have been included to illustrate the clinical severity of the DDE.

> I don't like the colour, I'm conscious about it, when I am talking I don't like showing them…. I'm actually quite bothered (boy, aged 15)

> I always wanted to change my teeth, they are like multi-coloured… I'm loads bothered (girl, aged 14) (Fig. 7.1)

> I've got some marks on the side of these two teeth, but they don't bother me (girl, aged 13)

Interestingly, DDE impacted most on individuals whose sense of self was defined by appearance and who depended on perceived approval from others about

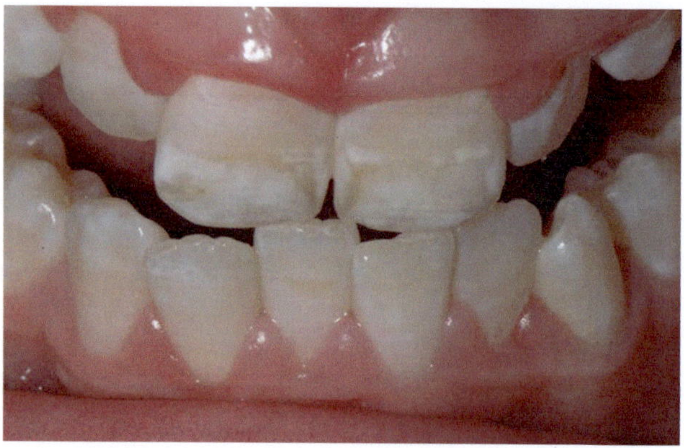

Fig. 7.2 Photograph of teeth of a participant with developmental enamel defects who said: "I'm happy with the way I am, it doesn't really matter what you look like, its personality" (girl, aged 12)

appearance. No association was found between gender, age, severity of DDE, and the reported impacts. However, this research was the first to identify that a sense of self may explain variation in the impact of DDE on young people. The following selected quotes illustrate how DDE were found to impact variably on the participants, in terms of how they felt about their own dental appearance.

> I don't want to look at myself in the mirror 'cos I know I'll look horrible…. (girl, aged 14)

> I'm happy with the way I am, it doesn't really matter what you look like, its personality. (girl, aged 12) (Fig. 7.2)

Another important finding was the degree to which children were teased or questioned about the marks on their teeth, particularly when new people were encountered. Again, there was considerable variation in how teasing and name-calling impacted on young people, which may have related to how much importance the individual placed on their appearance as a whole.

> I don't' like the thing on my tooth and I don't like my big ears. Whenever I get into an argument with someone that's the first thing they go on about (boy, aged 11)

> When people are being nasty they always say things about my teeth, I don't really care (girl, aged 12)

> Whenever I go on holiday or when I meet some new friends I don't know they say "I don't mean to be bad, but I think you've got something on your teeth there"… They thought I wasn't brushing them and stuff… (boy, aged 11)

Teasing and Bullying

Teasing, name-calling, and bullying are a common occurrence in childhood and adolescence. Lovegrove and Rumsey [26] found that over half of their sample of 654 British 11- to 14-year-olds had encountered appearance-related teasing or bullying. In a study of children with AI, 50 % reported being teased about their teeth

[16]. This figure concurs with findings from an earlier study of children with a range of DDE, where 56 % stated that they had been subject to unkind remarks about their teeth [22]. Although Marshman and colleagues [23] found variation in how teasing and name-calling impacted on young people, for some young people, being subject to teasing may be the motivation for seeking cosmetic treatment, and the clinician needs to be sensitive to such issues. However, young patients may be self-conscious and not always forthcoming about this matter, especially when meeting a dentist they do not know well. An empathetic approach is clearly needed, and the dentist should be able to direct patients to available support services, such as online anti-bullying resources (www.kidscape.org.uk).

The Impacts of Treatment for Enamel Defects

Dental Anxiety

The management of DDE encompasses a wide range of treatment regimens, which broadly aim to preserve tooth structure, prevent dental caries, reduce symptoms such as thermal hypersensitivity, and improve dental appearance. Some children face a lifetime of dental interventions in order to maintain their compromised dentition, and this may present considerable demands in terms of treatment compliance and costs for affected individuals and their families. Jälevik and Klingberg [33] highlighted the impacts of repeated treatment episodes for 9-year-old Swedish children with molar incisor hypomineralization (MIH). They found that children with MIH were more dentally anxious and were more likely to exhibit clinical behavior management problems than children in a control group. Interestingly, their longitudinal findings for the same group of children, 9 years later, revealed that although patients with MIH had poorer oral health (a significantly higher DMFT), they were no longer more dentally anxious then their non-MIH controls [34]. Clinical impressions suggest that children with AI may also be more dentally anxious than their peers [35], but this has yet to be evidenced by research findings. It is hypothesized that because these children frequently experience and anticipate oral pain from normally innocuous thermal, mechanical, and osmochemical stimuli, they understandably become more dentally anxious.

Psychosocial Outcomes

Patient-reported outcome measures are becoming more recognized within pediatric healthcare [36] but have yet to be well developed within dentistry. A recent Cochrane systematic review sought to compare clinical-reported and patient-reported outcomes (satisfaction with esthetics and sensitivity) following restorative care of children with AI [37]. Unfortunately, no studies met the inclusion criteria, but it was encouraging to see that the authors had recognized the need to seek children's views on what treatment outcomes were important to them.

To date, only one study appears to have considered the impact of treatment on young people with DDE [22]. This service evaluation sought the views of 67 young people, aged 7–16 years, who had received microabrasion and/or composite restorations on their upper incisors for a variety of visible enamel defects. Participants completed a simple 10-item questionnaire which was developed with service users. There was also a free text box for patients to write further comments. Prior to any intervention, children reported high levels of worry and embarrassment. However, following treatment, children said they felt happier and were more confident.

> I am a lot happier now, people don't pick on me (girl, aged 10)

> I cannot fault my treatment which has made me gain some confidence, which has helped me in this difficult year of exams (girl, aged 16)

Interestingly, the study also revealed unmet treatment expectations as some young people reported disappointment that their teeth "weren't perfect" after interventions. This finding clearly highlights the need for clinicians to communicate effectively and manage patient expectations more realistically at the outset of treatment. The media and celebrity culture may be influencing children to desire an unnaturally white and uniform dentition, which presents clinicians with ethical, financial, and clinical concerns.

> I was looking forward for seeing my teeth completely white but they were not completely white. It looked better than it was but they should have said that it wasn't going to do all my teeth white (boy, aged 14)

It is encouraging to see that a more recent study, conducted with children with AI, did seek young patients' expectations at the outset of treatment [16]. The authors asked 40 children what was the single most important thing they wanted from their course of treatment? The majority (63 %) stated that they hoped for an improvement in the color of their teeth, and 18 % said they wanted a better smile. For 10 %, a reduction in tooth sensitivity was the most important outcome.

Timing of Interventions

Another consideration is how the timing of any dental treatment, particularly for largely esthetic interventions, impacts on the individual. Clinical anecdote suggests that some children, who have been previously unconcerned about their dental appearance, are prompted to request treatment because of a significant social event (e.g., being a bridesmaid at a wedding) or change in their circumstances.

One study explored the experiences of 11- to 12-year-old children with a variety of visible facial and dental differences, including DDE, during their transition to secondary (high) school [17, 20, 22]. A 2-week diary was developed with children and incorporated both open and closed questions with space to include drawings.

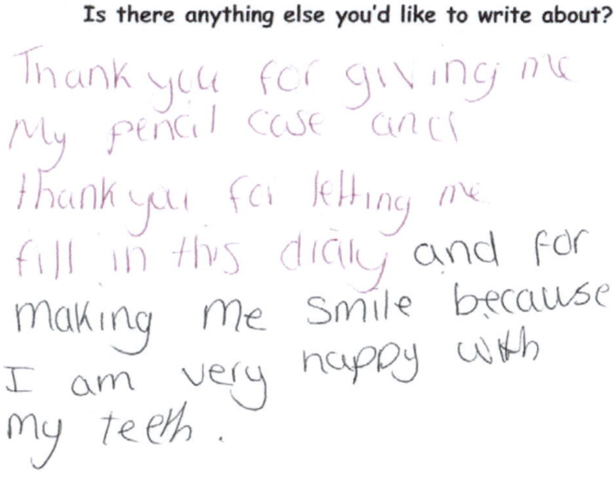
Is there anything else you'd like to write about?

Thank you for giving me my pencil case and thank you for letting me fill in this diary and for making me smile because I am very happy with my teeth.

Fig. 7.3 Extract from the diary of 11-year-old girl who had undergone microabrasion of her incisal opacities prior to moving to her new school

Children also completed the $CPQ_{11–14}$. Participants discussed a variety of aspects about the transition to secondary school including concerns about their appearance in their new social environment.

> I had like brown marks on the front two teeth, I didn't know what they were going to say about them…. it was a worry before I went to big school. (girl, aged 11)

Some children discussed their oral conditions such as cleft lip and how they dealt with questions from peers about it, while others reported having sought treatment to improve the appearance of enamel defects prior to starting secondary school (Fig. 7.3).

It should be noted, however, that heightened appearance-related concerns were not limited to oral conditions as some children stated that they had tried to lose weight, have their hair cut, or not to wear glasses prior to the transition. This enquiry demonstrated how impacts from DDE may be more or less important to a young person at different times during their life course, and dental care professionals should be sensitive to these issues when planning courses of treatment.

Another important consideration, relating to the provision of dental treatment, is how this may impact on a child's school attendance and social activities. The need for frequent dental visits, often at a specialist practice some distance from home, is likely to have a social impact on the child and their family. However, our review of the literature failed to reveal any studies in this area.

In general, the evidence base is lacking to support the psychosocial benefits of DDE-related treatment for young people. This should be a priority for future research as it becomes increasingly important that treatments are justified and evaluated in terms of patient benefit. Longitudinal studies are paramount to consider both the short- and long-term psychosocial effects of different dental interventions and thereby develop and safeguard services for young people with DDE.

Social Judgments in Relation to Enamel Defects

Appearance-Related Judgments

There is a wealth of literature to support the association between an individual's appearance, especially facial appearance, and how they are perceived by others [38]. A fascinating study by Dion showed that children who were considered less attractive than other children would be viewed as more likely by an adult to have committed a misdemeanor and were viewed as less honest [39]. The seminal work by Langlois and colleagues [40] also demonstrated that attractive children were rated more positively for a number of personal attributes than those considered unattractive. Regrettably, we live in a society where appearance does matter, and those who look different may elicit negative judgments which have important social consequences, including even future job prospects.

Children's Views of Other Children with Enamel Defects

The first study to consider how a child's dental appearance influenced how their peers and adults viewed them was conducted by Shaw [41]. Children, depicted in photographs, as having well-aligned teeth and normal facial appearance were judged to be better looking, more desirable as friends, more intelligent, and less likely to behave aggressively than children with a malocclusion or cleft lip.

More recently, a similar methodology was employed to determine whether, or not, young people made value judgments, or ascribed certain social attributes, to other young people with visible enamel defects [21]. Focus groups were first conducted with children aged 11 to 16 years to identify what terminology they used, or judgments they made, in relation to photographs of teeth with a range of DDE. Two common themes emerged from these discussions with participants perceiving that people with DDE were "lazy" or "did not care about their appearance" (Fig. 7.4).

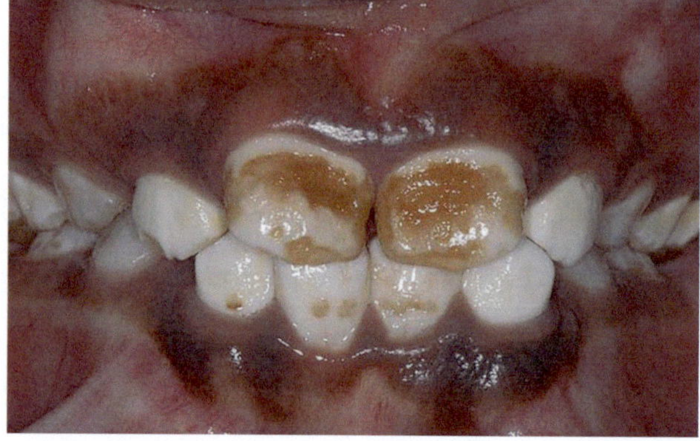

Fig. 7.4 Children's judgments relating to this photograph of a child with severe dental fluorosis included: [this person] "has no personal hygiene," "has eaten too much syrup," and "is lazy"

The investigators then recruited 547 school children, aged 11–12 and 14–15 years, to rate full-face photographs of a boy and girl using a social attribute questionnaire that had been previously developed with young people. The 11 social attributes included: kind, rude, clever, honest, cares about appearance, careful, lazy, confident, helpful, stupid, and naughty. Half the participants were shown photographs of the boy and girl with normal teeth, and half were shown digitally modified photographs of the same children with a visible enamel defect affecting one upper incisor. The key finding was that young people did make negative social judgments on the basis of DDE. Age and socioeconomic status did not have an effect on raters' scores, but girls were more positive in their assessment than boys. Affected individuals may be unfairly judged by others which may, in turn, impact on their self-esteem, social interactions, and life prospects.

Summary and Clinical Implications

This brief review of the literature, albeit an emerging literature, suggests that having a DDE can impact on children and young people in a variety of ways. Generic oral health-related quality of life questionnaires have provided conflicting findings, but qualitative enquires have given a richer and more meaningful insight into the range and severity of psychosocial impacts. Appearance-related impacts are foremost with some children reporting embarrassment, upset, and reluctance to smile or show their teeth in normal social interactions. In addition, some children may experience dental hypersensitivity as well as compromised esthetics, which are likely to have negative impacts on daily activities. For young patients requiring extensive dental treatment, there is the potential to develop dental anxiety. Studies have also shown that some children with DDE are subject to dental appearance-related teasing and may incur negative social judgments from their peers. Most of the research to date has been conducted on the impact of DDE in the permanent dentition with little knowledge about the nature or severity of the impact of DDE on younger children.

Some individuals with a visible difference cope better than others but the reasons for their resilience have not been fully elucidated. This observation is supported by the finding that there is no simple correlation between the severity of the enamel defect and the resultant impact. Further research, in collaboration with social science experts, is indicated to explore these complex and dynamic relationships, throughout childhood and adolescence.

The "take-home" message for clinicians is that children and young people with DDE require an empathetic and insightful approach. Every effort should be made to provide timely and aesthetic care, which addresses the young patient's individual concerns and circumstances. However, unrealistic treatment expectations may be encountered, and these need to be met with good communication and appropriate support. It is important that robust pediatric patient-reported outcome measures are developed for future use, so that we can be sure that our treatment is actually helping to reduce the psychosocial impacts of having an enamel defect.

References

1. Do LG, Spencer A. Oral health-related quality of life of children by dental caries and fluorosis experience. J Public Health Dent. 2007;67(3):132–9.
2. Arrow P. Child oral health-related quality of life (COHQoL), enamel defects of the first permanent molars and caries experience among children in Western Australia. Community Dent Health. 2013;30(3):183–8.
3. Bendo C, Paiva S, Varni J, Vale M. Oral health-related quality of life and traumatic dental injuries in Brazilian adolescents. Community Dent Oral Epidemiol. 2014;42(3):216–23.
4. Eslami N, Majidi MR, Aliakbarian M, Hasanzadeh N. Oral health-related quality of life in children with cleft lip and palate. J Craniofac Surg. 2013;24(4):e340–3.
5. Kotecha S, Turner PJ, Dietrich T, Dhopatkar A. The impact of tooth agenesis on oral health-related quality of life in children. J Orthod. 2013;40(2):122–9.
6. Scapini A, Feldens CA, Ardenghi TM, Kramer PF. Malocclusion impacts adolescents' oral health-related quality of life. Angle Orthod. 2013;83(3):512–8.
7. Hall M, Gibson B, James A, Rodd HD. Children's experiences of participation in the cleft lip and palate care pathway. Int J Paediatr Dent. 2012;22(6):442–50.
8. Gilchrist F, Rodd HD, Deery C, Marshman Z. Involving children in research, audit and service evaluation. Br Dent J. 2013;214(11):577–82.
9. Jokovic A, Locker D, Guyatt G. Short forms of the Child Perceptions Questionnaire for 11–14-year-old children (CPQ(11–14)): development and initial evaluation. Health Qual Life Outcomes. 2006;4:4.
10. Jokovic A, Locker D, Stephens M, Kenny D, Tompson B, Guyatt G. Validity and reliability of a questionnaire for measuring child oral-health-related quality of life. J Dent Res. 2002;81(7):459–63.
11. Jokovic A, Locker D, Tompson B, Guyatt G. Questionnaire for measuring oral health-related quality of life in eight- to ten-year-old children. Pediatr Dent. 2004;26(6):512–8.
12. Broder HL, McGrath C, Cisneros GJ. Questionnaire development: face validity and item impact testing of the child oral health impact profile. Community Dent Oral Epidemiol. 2007;35:8–19.
13. Gherunpong S, Tsakos G, Sheiham A. Developing and evaluating an oral health-related quality of life index for children; the CHILD-OIDP. Community Dent Health. 2004;21(2):161–9.
14. Astrom AN, Mashoto K. Determinants of self-rated oral health status among school children in northern Tanzania. Int J Paediatr Dent. 2002;12(2):90–100.
15. Michel-Crosato E, Biazevic MGH, Crosato E. Relationship between dental fluorosis and quality of life: a population based study. Braz Oral Res. 2005;19(2):150–5.
16. Parekh S, Almehateb M, Cunningham SJ. How do children with amelogenesis imperfecta feel about their teeth? Int J Paediatr Dent. 2014;24(5):326–35.
17. Rodd HD, Marshman Z, Porritt J, Bradbury J, Baker SR. Oral health-related quality of life of children in relation to dental appearance and educational transition. Br Dent J. 2011;211(2):E4.
18. Rodd HD, Marshman Z, Porritt J, Bradbury J, Baker SR. Psychosocial predictors of children's oral health-related quality of life during transition to secondary school. Qual Life Res. 2012;21(4):707–16.
19. Coffield KD, Phillips C, Brady M, Roberts MW, Strauss RP, Wright JT. The psychosocial impact of developmental dental defects in people with hereditary amelogenesis imperfecta. J Am Dent Assoc. 2005;136(5):620–30.
20. Marshman Z, Baker SR, Bradbury J, Hall MJ, Rodd HD. The psychosocial impact of oral conditions during transition to secondary education. Eur J Paediatr Dent. 2009;10(4):176–80.
21. Craig S. How children view other children with enamel defects. MPhil thesis. Sheffield: University of Sheffield; 2013.
22. Rodd HD, Abdul-Karim A, Yesudian G, O'Mahony J, Marshman Z. Seeking children's perspectives in the management of visible enamel defects. Int J Paediatr Dent. 2011; 21(2):89–95.

23. Marshman Z, Gibson B, Robinson PG. The impact of developmental defects of enamel on young people in the UK. Community Dent Oral Epidemiol. 2009;37(1):45–57.
24. Vargas-Ferreira F, Ardenghi TM. Developmental enamel defects and their impact on child oral health-related quality of life. Braz Oral Res. 2011;25(6):531–7.
25. Pope AW, Ward J. Self-perceived facial appearance and psychosocial adjustment in preadolescents with craniofacial anomalies. Cleft Palate Craniofac J. 1997;34(5):396–401.
26. Lovegrove E, Rumsey N. Ignoring it doesn't make it stop: adolescents, appearance, and bullying. Cleft Palate Craniofac J. 2005;42(1):33–44.
27. Helderman WHV, Mkasabuni E. Impact of dental fluorosis on the perception of well-being in an endemic fluorosis area in Tanzania. Community Dent Oral Epidemiol. 1993;21(4):243–4.
28. Chankanka O, Levy SM, Warren JJ, Chalmers JM. A literature review of aesthetic perceptions of dental fluorosis and relationships with psychosocial aspects/oral health-related quality of life. Community Dent Oral Epidemiol. 2010;38(2):97–109.
29. Sujak SL, Abdul Kadir R, Dom TN. Esthetic perception and psychosocial impact of developmental enamel defects among Malaysian adolescents. J Oral Sci. 2004;46(4):221–6.
30. Robinson PG, Nalweyiso N, Busingye J, Whitworth J. Subjective impacts of dental caries and fluorosis in rural Ugandan children. Community Dent Health. 2005;22(4):231–6.
31. Locker D. Disparities in oral health-related quality of life in a population of Canadian children. Community Dent Oral Epidemiol. 2007;35(5):348–56.
32. Poulsen S, Gjorup H, Haubek D, Haukali G, Hintze H, Lovschall H, et al. Amelogenesis imperfecta – a systematic literature review of associated dental and oro-facial abnormalities and their impact on patients. Acta Odontol Scand. 2008;66(4):193–9.
33. Jalevik B, Klingberg GA. Dental treatment, dental fear and behaviour management problems in children with severe enamel hypomineralization of their permanent first molars. Int J Paediatr Dent. 2002;12(1):24–32.
34. Jalevik B, Klingberg G. Treatment outcomes and dental anxiety in 18-year-olds with MIH, comparisons with healthy controls – a longitudinal study. Int J Paediatr Dent. 2012;22(2):85–91.
35. McDonald S, Arkutu N, Malik K, Gadhia K, McKaig S. Managing the paediatric patient with amelogenesis imperfecta. Br Dent J. 2012;212(9):425–8.
36. Bevans KB, Riley AW, Moon J, Forrest CB. Conceptual and methodological advances in child-reported outcomes measurement. Expert Rev Pharmacoecon Outcomes Res. 2010;10(4):385–96.
37. Dashash M, Yeung CA, Jamous I, Blinkhorn A. Interventions for the restorative care of amelogenesis imperfecta in children and adolescents. Cochrane Database Syst Rev. 2013;6:CD007157.
38. Zebrowitz L, Montepare J. Social psychological face perception: why appearance matters. Soc Pers Psychol Compass. 2008;2:1497–517.
39. Dion K. Physical attractiveness and evaluation of children's transgressions. J Pers Soc Psychol. 1972;24(2):207–13.
40. Langlois JH, Kalakanis L, Rubenstein AJ, Larson A, Hallam M, Smoot M. Maxims or myths of beauty? A meta-analytic and theoretical review. Psychol Bull. 2000;126(3):390–423.
41. Shaw WC. The influence of children's dentofacial appearance on their social attractiveness as judged by peers and lay adults. Am J Orthod Dentofacial Orthop. 1981;79(4):399–415.

Examination and Treatment Planning for Hypomineralized and/or Hypoplastic Teeth

8

Bernadette K. Drummond and Winifred Harding

Abstract

When children present with teeth with developmental defects of enamel (DDE), achieving long-term successful outcomes for the teeth is dependent on establishing a diagnosis of the problems and on immediate, short- and longer-term treatment planning. Good records (medical and dental history as well as clinical radiographic, photographic, and histologic examination) that are available for successive clinicians who treat the child are also important. It is also important to consider referral for medical evaluation if it is thought the defects are related to a general systemic or genetic condition that has not been investigated. This chapter provides guidance on the process of examination required to establish a diagnosis and possible treatment options including the impact on the developing occlusion when those options may involve extractions.

Introduction

It can be difficult to diagnose if enamel is hypomineralized or hypoplastic and to establish how the appearance, color, and position of defects may affect the quality of the enamel. Currently there is no recommended clinical charting for developmental defects of enamel (DDE) that reflects the diagnosis and indicates how the teeth should be managed. Establishing a diagnosis can identify potential long-term issues including the impact of the type of defect on enamel bonding. There is also not a good evidence base for restorative management or bonding protocols for DDE-affected teeth.

B.K. Drummond, BDS, MS, PhD (✉)
Department of Oral Sciences, Faculty of Dentistry, University of Otago,
310 Great King Street, PO Box 647, Dunedin 9054, New Zealand
e-mail: bernadette.drummond@otago.ac.nz

W. Harding, BDS, MDS
Department of Oral Sciences, Discipline of Orthodontics, Faculty of Dentistry,
University of Otago, 310 Great King Street, PO Box 647, Dunedin, New Zealand
e-mail: winifred@southnet.co.nz

© Springer-Verlag Berlin Heidelberg 2015
B.K. Drummond, N. Kilpatrick (eds.), *Planning and Care for Children and Adolescents with Dental Enamel Defects: Etiology, Research and Contemporary Management*, DOI 10.1007/978-3-662-44800-7_8

Despite many papers describing the structure and composition of defective enamel (see Chaps. 5 and 6), there is still limited understanding of how enamel with decreased mineral and/or with increased protein content can be successfully managed with currently available restorative procedures. Understanding the diagnosis will allow the immediate needs to be considered including management of sensitivity, poor esthetics, and posteruptive breakdown (PEB). Because the defects are usually diagnosed in young children, once the immediate problems have been managed, an intermediate management plan should be developed to preserve the teeth until permanent restorations can be placed, often over a decade later. Early management may include using preventive materials to decrease caries risk and sensitivity, masking defects to improve appearance, and temporarily and/or permanently restoring hypoplastic defects. It can seem tempting to extract teeth when only one or a few teeth are affected, but full assessment of occlusal development is important to consider orthodontic treatment needs. Young patients have a wide range of coping skills, and sedation or general anesthesia may be required to optimize outcomes. There are also financial implications. While funding may be available to support dental treatment during childhood, it may not be as accessible in early adulthood when definitive restorations are planned. Long-term planning should therefore also take in to consideration the ability of the child/family to afford anticipated treatment. Families require a significant amount of knowledge of the problems associated with DDE to understand that the affected teeth will require a lifetime of dental care even when they remain caries and erosion free. This chapter considers what should be included in the examination, diagnosis, and treatment planning when children present with teeth with DDE.

Description of Enamel Defects

The appearances of DDE have been described in previous chapters (Chaps. 1, 2, 3, and 5) but are summarized again in Table 8.1. While the descriptors have been mainly developed for epidemiological studies, they are useful clinically to help diagnose the type of defect.

Table 8.1 Descriptions of enamel defects that have been used in epidemiological studies

Type of defect	Extent of defects	Diffuse opacities	Demarcated opacities
Normal	Less than one third	Diffuse lines	White cream
Diffuse opacity	Between one and two thirds	Diffuse patchy	Yellow brown
Demarcated opacity	At least two thirds	Diffuse confluent	
Hypoplasia		Staining	
Hypoplasia pits		Pits	
Hypoplasia grooves		Loss of enamel	
Hypoplasia, missing enamel, discoloration			
Any other			

Clinical History

As many opacities and hypoplastic defects appear to have no obvious cause, a careful and accurate history can pinpoint the timing in relation to possible associated medical events when the defects may have occurred. There will often be a history of repeated attempts to restore teeth with DDE or of a child who is often described as uncooperative. This suggests that because of the sensitivity of affected teeth, children have been more anxious, and local anesthesia has not been successful [1]. In older children, first molars in molar incisor hypomineralization (MIH) may have already been extracted. Table 8.2 summarizes the information that is useful in the clinical history.

The problems, signs, and symptoms given by the child should be recorded. It can sometimes be difficult to elicit concerns or a pain history from younger children but suitable questions often help identify the issues, as suggested in Table 8.3 and described in Chap. 7.

Table 8.2 Information from the clinical history

Information	Relevance
Family history	May suggest a genetic cause (Chap. 5)
Birth history	Neonatal events (Chaps. 1, 2, and 4)
Pregnancy history	Pregnancy history and mother's health
Childhood systemic illnesses	Timing of childhood illnesses (Chap. 4)
Drug and medication history	Evidence of drugs, medication, and supplements affecting enamel development (Chaps. 2 and 3)
Allergies	Enamel defects in with conditions such as celiac disease (Chap. 4)
Hypocalcemia	Associated with prematurity, Vitamin D deficiency, and maternal diabetes (Chaps. 1 and 2)
Nutritional problems	Exclusive breast feeding beyond 6 months, Vitamin D deficiency (Chaps. 1 and 2)
Caries history	From the primary dentition. If only second primary molars restored – suggestive these teeth may have had DDE

Table 8.3 Children's history indicating teeth problems

Question/comment	Explanation
It hurts to brush my teeth	Teeth are too sensitive
My teacher says I don't clean my teeth properly	Many people think opacities and other DDE are due to a lack of brushing
Mother describes child never smiling	Suggests that children do not like their appearance
My friends make fun of me	Demonstrates a social problem for the child
My teeth have sharp edges	An issue for children with hypoplastic or fractured enamel
Can't eat ice cream	Indicates a significant sensitivity problem
Parents say child eats slowly or refuses some foods	Suggests sensitive teeth and food trapping

Clinical Examination

The clinical examination should note the sites, size, and appearance of DDE on individual primary and/or permanent teeth. This can help to differentiate between isolated insults during development or a genetic- or systemic-related problem that has affected all the teeth. DDE in selected primary teeth can indicate a potential problem in permanent teeth. Developmental defects of the primary second molar alone are suggestive of hypomineralized second primary molars (HSPM) which are predictive of MIH as discussed in Chap. 3. Developmental defects that affect all the primary teeth may indicate a more generalized impact in the permanent dentition (Chaps. 4 and 5). The texture and color of the enamel indicate the presence of hypoplasia and/or hypomineralization. The darker the color, particularly in MIH, the higher the enamel protein content, indicating increased risk of cohesive failure of bonded restorations [2]. Texture can be determined by gently running a probe across the surface. Enamel that is opaque may have a relatively smooth texture reflecting the fact that the surface enamel has mineralized further after eruption. However it is important to remember that from the bonding perspective, the subsurface is still hypomineralized. Color and texture will partly determine the restorative approaches. In hypomineralized enamel without hypoplasia or breakdown, attempts can be made to improve the appearance using microabrasion with and without bleaching or possibly resin infiltration. This is discussed further in Chap. 11. Areas of posteruptive breakdown or hypoplasia should be noted as well as the position of normal enamel that can be utilized to optimize bonding and achieve a sound marginal seal for restorations. In most MIH-affected first permanent molars, there is a band of relatively normal enamel at or below the gingival margin as shown in Fig. 8.1. This allows for good permanent crown margins in late adolescence once pulps have matured and teeth have erupted to provide an acceptable crown height. The challenge in a young child is how to achieve protection of the crowns and pulps of affected teeth until late adolescence (Chaps. 9 and 11 discuss management options).

Care should be taken when diagnosing caries. What appears to be caries visually may be found to be sound dentine with posteruptive enamel breakdown after the surface has been cleaned and dried. This is important as non-carious dentine should

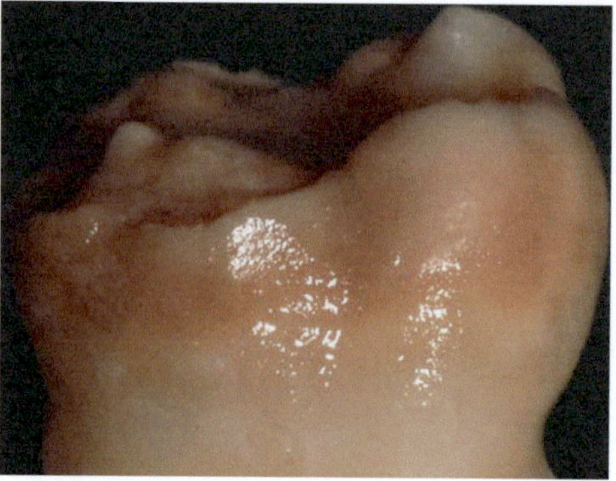

Fig. 8.1 View of extracted lower first molar crown showing "normal" enamel at or below the gingival margin (Courtesy of Dr. Rami Farah)

be preserved when restoring hypomineralized teeth and so consideration needs to be given to dentine, as well as enamel bonding in the restorative technique. This is discussed further in Chap. 11.

Radiographic Examination

Panoramic radiography is essential to establish the presence or absence of all permanent teeth and to assess the stage of development of the dentition. This is very important if extractions are being considered as part of the management plan. Calcification of the second premolar crowns will be evident in the early mixed dentition. However, calcification of the third molar crowns does not begin until 7–10 years of age, and this should be taken into account when taking radiographs and planning treatment (Fig. 8.2). The developmental stages of each tooth and anomalies in shape and size as well as in eruption paths should be recorded to consider the possibility of other associated conditions. Bitewing radiographs can help determine if caries is occurring alongside hypomineralization when the shapes of radiolucent lesions are compared and the dentine is examined (Fig. 8.3).

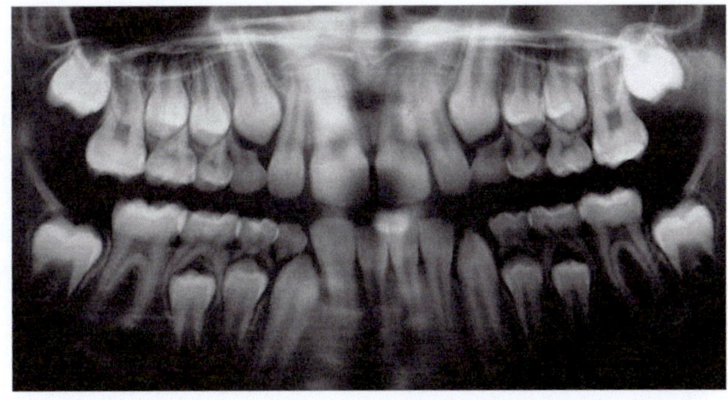

Fig. 8.2 Panoramic radiograph of a 9-year-old boy with severe hypomineralization of the upper first molars. Third molars are not evident

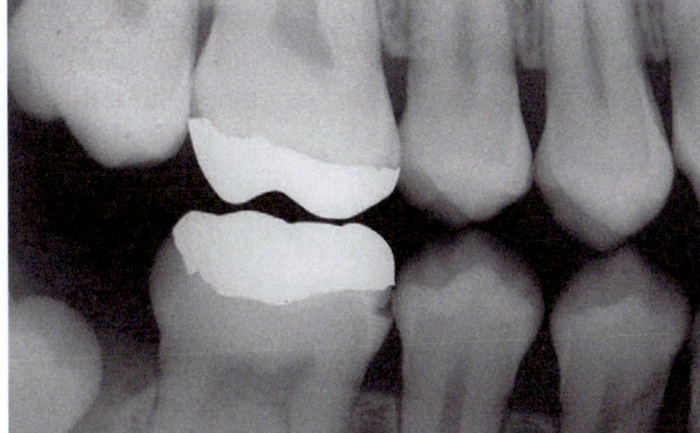

Fig. 8.3 Right posterior bitewing radiograph of an 11-year-old girl with gold overlays on the upper and lower right first molars. Note the hypomineralized enamel on the mesial and distal surfaces and suspected enamel caries on the mesial of the lower first molar

Histological Examination

When a systemic or genetic cause for the DDE is suspected, it is recommended that any available teeth be examined histologically. The histological appearance will help to determine a more accurate diagnosis and provide the clinician with a better understanding of the condition and likely behavior of the tissues when planning restorative care. Histology can be carried out on exfoliated primary teeth or ideally on permanent teeth if they become available.

Medical Examination

Teeth with DDE may be associated with a systemic condition or a syndrome. Occasionally a problem has not been diagnosed, and where this is suspected, children should be referred to a pediatrician with the relevant orofacial history and concerns. It is useful to include copies of radiographs or histology reports which can be added to the general medical record. Where a genetic cause is determined, advice may be sought from a geneticist to determine the genes involved or to give the child and parents more information about the inheritance pattern.

Assessment of Growth and Development

Early assessment of growth and development is essential in children who present with DDE. Where possible, an orthodontic opinion should be included in the assessment, particularly if there is an associated malocclusion and/or consideration is being given to extracting first permanent molars because of their poor prognosis. The implications of long-term restorative needs have to be weighed up against possible outcomes in the developing dentition if teeth are removed, particularly if there is a malocclusion that will worsen with early loss of teeth. It is important that the clinician informs the orthodontist of the long-term prognosis of the teeth including the likelihood of complex restorative care throughout adulthood. In cases of defects with severe posteruptive breakdown (PEB) or hypoplasia with associated malocclusion, positioning of teeth is important for future prosthodontic management. The primary care dentist or pediatric dentist can play an important role in coordinating prosthodontic and orthodontic evaluations to determine the best long-term plan. Extraction of teeth may at first seem a useful solution, but careful planning is needed to limit later occlusion problems. It is important to consider caries risk, as extracting teeth in children who have a history of caries and are likely to remain at risk may not be a sensible solution for the whole dentition in the long term. This is particularly important if subsequent fixed appliance orthodontic treatment is going to be needed to close extraction spaces, upright second molars, or correct an existing malocclusion. Space analysis can predict relationships of the teeth to the arches and space available.

Table 8.4 Information from growth and development assessment

Extraorally	Skeletal pattern
	Face height
	TMJ
	Symmetry
	Lip competency
Intraorally	Permanent and primary molar relationships
	Canine relationships (primary or permanent depending on age)
	Position and inclination of canines
	Crossbite with/without displacement
	Position of midlines
	Inclination of upper and lower incisors
	Overjet and overbite
	Crowding or spacing of the teeth
	Curve of Spee
Teeth	Teeth – present and unerupted (radiographs)
	Caries – clinical and radiographic
	Teeth defects clinical and radiographic
	Other anomalies – missing, supernumerary, malformed teeth
Space analysis	Amount or lack of space should be estimated
Photographs	Important record for longer-term recording of the changes
Study models	Important record of the developing occlusion

Information to Be Recorded

Because children with DDE will face ongoing treatment needs, it is important to produce good records that can be used throughout childhood and adolescence. Table 8.4 suggests the clinical and orofacial developmental features that should be recorded.

Treatment Planning

Treatment planning for children with DDE will determine the stages of treatment to optimize long-term survival of the teeth [3]. Many children with DDE do not cope well with dental treatment. This will play a significant role in the decision-making process as many options require the child/adolescent to cope with complex long-term restorative and/or orthodontic care. Planning should optimize the timing of treatment and minimize the need for repeated procedures when sedation or general anesthesia is needed. Financial considerations will also impact on treatment choices and need to be acknowledged both for short- and longer-term treatment plans. Table 8.5 summarizes possible management options in the immediate, short-term and long-term management of teeth with enamel defects.

Table 8.5 Short-, medium-, and long-term management options

Immediate	Explanation
Controlling sensitivity	Allows good oral hygiene and child can manage treatment (Chap. 9)
Preventing dental caries	Teeth with DDE are more susceptible to faster caries progression in hypomineralized or hypoplastic teeth (Chap. 9)
Temporary restorations	Useful in the short term but important to avoid repeated efforts to restore or seal teeth to avoid child developing dental anxiety
Improving enamel	Long-term protection, improved bonding, decrease risk of fracture
Improving aesthetics	Very important in the anterior region to improve child self-esteem
Medium term (3–10 years)	**Explanation**
Controlling sensitivity	Needed until permanent restorations are provided in molar teeth unless temporary coverage has been possible
Preventing dental caries	Home prevention, frequent recalls, professional fluoride treatments, and sealing where appropriate (Chap. 9)
Restoring defects	Temporary restorations need regular monitoring and resealing (Chap. 11)
Managing pulp health	Dentine and enamel should be sealed to protect pulp and allow maturation. Pulpal exposure or infection can be managed with a range of procedures that can maintain the teeth until long-term solutions are decided [4]
Acceptable aesthetics	Important in childhood and adolescence for confidence (Chap. 7)
Temporary crowns	Stainless steel crowns are an excellent solution for primary and permanent molars. Polymethyl methacrylate (resin) crowns provide acceptable outcomes in dentitions with AI [5]. Both support the occlusion until early adulthood (Chaps. 10 and 11)
Extraction of teeth Orthodontic care	Extraction of teeth is an option in some dentitions. Important to consider timing and possible need for associated orthodontic care [7].
Long term	**Explanation**
Cast metal overlays	Cast metal overlays can be successful in molars with moderate hypomineralized defects and PEB or wear (Chap. 11)
Ceramic onlays	Ceramic onlays may be considered for molar teeth. Unacceptable wear of opposing teeth with immature enamel may occur [5]
Veneers	Porcelain veneers provide excellent aesthetics anteriorly. Not recommended until complete eruption has occurred in late adolescence or early adulthood (Chap. 11)
Crowns	Several options available when enough tooth tissue to support a crown. Success is dependent on temporary care that is provided through childhood and adolescence (Chap. 11)

Practical Management When Extractions Are Being Considered

When planning the longer-term management of hypomineralized or hypoplastic teeth, an orthodontic consultation is important to inform the child and parents of possible outcomes for the occlusion and what can be done if teeth are extracted.

It is important that the orthodontist is aware of the prognosis of the teeth so that they can include this in their assessment of the risks and benefits of possible orthodontic options. As it is not always possible to involve an orthodontist, the following is a guide when planning extraction of first permanent molars. It allows appropriate information to be given to the child and parents. It is recommended that details be carefully recorded and given to the family in written form. This includes clinical and radiographic details and photographs. It can help answer questions about the treatment that may come many years later. Details that should be recorded include:

1. Are teeth restorable with good long-term prognosis and without repeated restorations?
2. Are the third molars developing? Are there other missing teeth?
3. Are the second molars developing normally with acceptable eruption paths to erupt into functional occlusion? What are their stages of development?
4. Are all the premolars developing normally with normal eruption paths?
5. Are other teeth hypomineralized? Is this a generalized problem?
6. If there is crowding, what impact will the extractions have?
7. What is the anterior occlusion including overbite and overjet? Will the overbite be acceptable if molars are extracted or will it increase? Is there a lip trap?
8. What is the facial growth pattern?

These questions and the following information provide guidance on planning whether to extract or keep first permanent molars with defects. There are generally four possible options:

1. Extract immediately if age and stage of development are appropriate or the tooth is not restorable, even temporarily
2. Delay extraction to optimize the eruption of surrounding teeth
3. Delay extraction until done as part of orthodontic treatment
4. Keep and plan the path to permanent restoration of the tooth/teeth

Outcomes of Extraction of First Molars

Where conditions are favorable, satisfactory space closure can be achieved when first molar extractions are done in children and young adults [8–10]. Williams and Hosila [11] noted that extraction of first permanent molars was associated with less effect on the profile and significantly more likelihood of third molars erupting than with premolar extractions. First molar extraction will not always relieve crowding posteriorly, but improvements in third molar eruption have been reported [6, 12, 13]. In the majority of children with early loss of permanent first molars before 12 years of age, third molar development appears to be accelerated on the side of the extraction [14]. Figure 8.4 a–c shows the outcome of extracting a single lower molar at a time to optimize eruption of the second permanent molar.

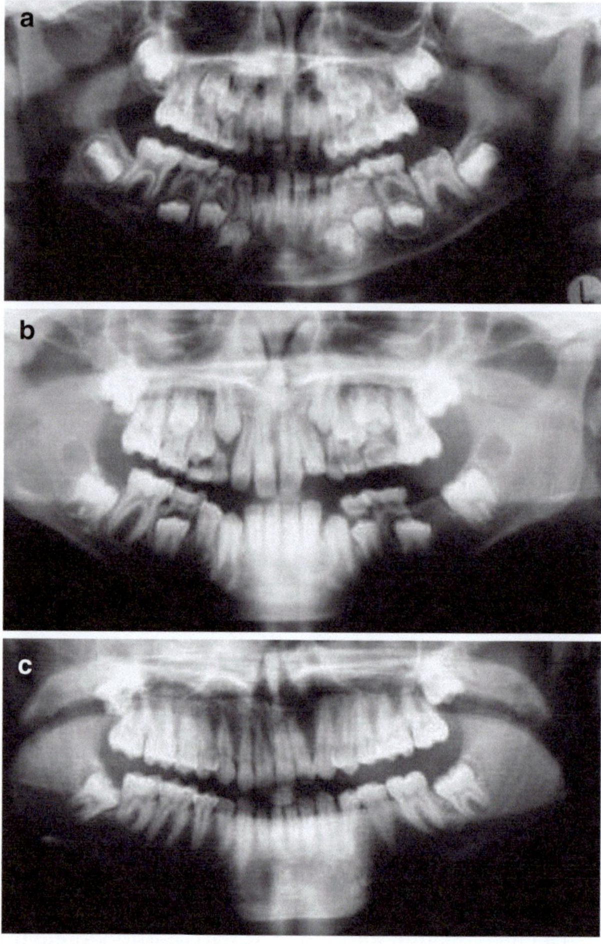

Fig. 8.4 Panoramic radiographs showing (**a**) a broken down lower left first molar, (**b**) 2 years following extraction, (**c**) 9 years following extraction showing good position of early erupting lower left third molar

The following can be considered:

1. In dentitions with excess space in the arches, extractions may leave permanent spaces or orthodontic treatment may be needed to close unacceptable spacing.
2. When molars are extracted in one quadrant only, overeruption of the opposing molar or occlusal interferences may occur. Compensating extractions (i.e., removal of the opposing tooth) are not always advised. Balancing extractions (i.e., removal of the contralateral tooth) can be considered after the available space and anterior occlusion are taken into account. In some instances a balancing extraction may be a premolar on the opposite side especially where the opposite molar is not compromised. There can be a risk of midline shift when only one molar is extracted [15].
3. When a lower first molar is extracted, occlusal forces can influence mesial and lingual tilting of the second molar because of the thinner lingual plate. Lingual positioning may result in a scissor bite or nonworking side interferences that can

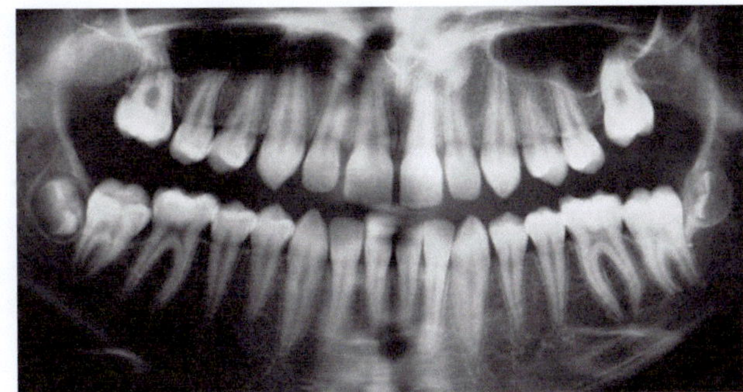

Fig. 8.5 Panoramic radiograph of an adolescent who had both upper first molars extracted 2 years previously

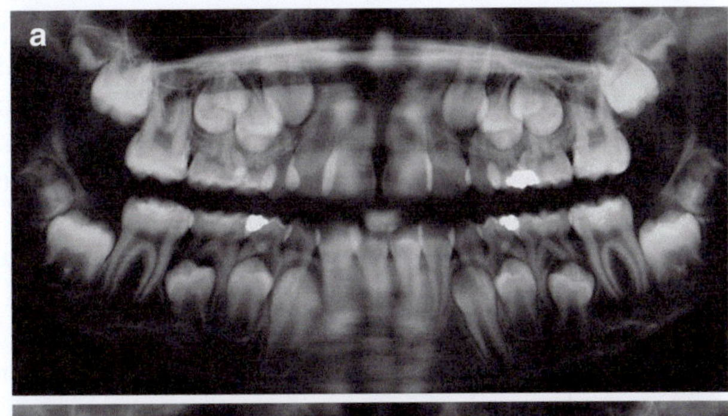

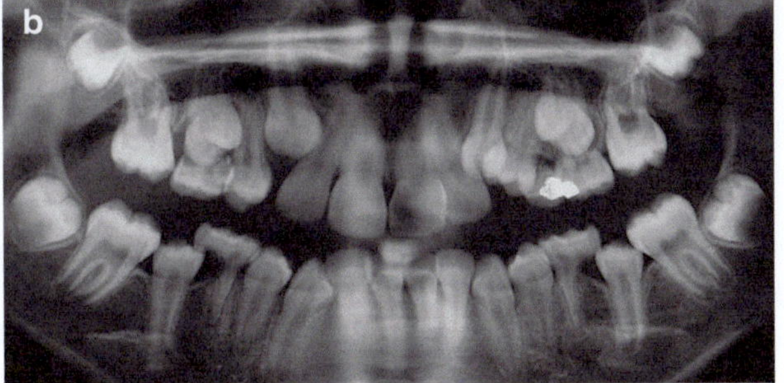

Fig. 8.6 (**a**) Panoramic of 9-year-old female with an orthodontic plan to have all first molars extracted (severe hypomineralization). Note positions of lower second premolars. (**b**) Panoramic 3 years after the extractions. Note eruption paths of lower second premolars

cause unwanted tooth wear. Poor interproximal contacts can lead to food impaction and difficulty in cleaning. This is less likely to occur with an upper first molar extraction, as the upper second molar will usually erupt into a good position as long as the second molar is unerupted at the time of the extraction as illustrated in Fig. 8.5.

4. Early extraction of first permanent molars before 8 years-of-age may result in distal drifting, tilting, and rotation of unerupted second premolars even in well-aligned arches. In severe ectopic eruption, the second premolar may impact against the second molar as it erupts. Where a distal eruption path of the second premolar is detected, the second primary molar could be extracted at the same time as the first molar extraction to encourage a vertical eruption path for the premolar (Fig. 8.6a, b).

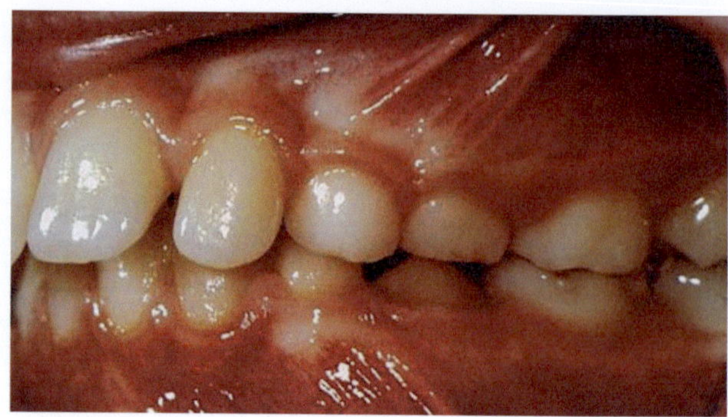

Fig. 8.7 Patient in mixed dentition illustrating deep bite which would probably worsen if the first molars were extracted

5. An increase in overbite can occur following the early extraction of first molars. Retroclination of the lower incisors worsens in children with previously proclined upper incisors and increased overjet [16]. In children with decreased facial height, crowded lower anteriors, or a deep overbite, early extraction of the first molars is contraindicated without management to prevent further problems in the anterior occlusion (Fig. 8.6).

6. Where there is a skeletal or dental malocclusion, extractions may be timed to utilize space to correct the malocclusion:

   (a) In a class II occlusion with maxillary protrusion, upper first molar spaces may be required for anterior teeth retraction.

   (b) With a lower lip trap and increased overjet, extraction of lower first molars can result in lower incisor retroclination which may increase overjet and complicate treatment (Fig. 8.7).

   (c) In bimaxillary protrusion, first molar extraction spaces may be required for anterior retraction.

   (d) In severe crowding, first molar extraction spaces may be required to alleviate the crowding.

   (e) Distal drift of the lower premolars may occur after lower first molar extractions to allow improvement in alignment of the anterior teeth where the overjet and overbite are acceptable, but this rarely occurs in the upper arch.

   (f) In class III malocclusions, lower first molar extraction spaces may be needed for lower anterior teeth retraction.

   (g) With maxillary constriction, the first molars may be needed for expansion devices.

   (h) With a skeletal anterior open bite, early extraction of first molars may be advantageous as part of orthodontic management.

7. To optimize the eruption of second molars into first molar positions, the timing of extractions, particularly the lower, is important. Ideal timing is usually around 9–10 years of age, when the bifurcation dentine of the second molar is mineralizing with the beginning of root formation [17, 18] (Fig. 8.2). Temporary measures may be necessary to retain the teeth in an infection- and pain-free state until the ideal time for the extractions. This timing will encourage the eruption of the second molar (often early) into contact with the second premolar in an uncrowded dentition.

Conclusion

This chapter has covered aspects of clinical and radiographic examination and treatment planning for children with DDE. It has provided some guidance when considering options to extract teeth that have DDE. Careful planning that includes the management of sensitivity and esthetics will help the child to care for their teeth and develop skills to cope with dental treatment. An important aspect is the need to keep good records of both the original diagnoses and initial treatments as teeth with defects will require long-term treatment and records can be given to successive clinicians to aid in planning further care. Although young children may be difficult to manage, they deserve even more attention when they have DDE because the care given in the early permanent dentition can have a profound impact on the outcomes for the life of the teeth and on the child's ability to continue seeking dental care.

References

1. Jälevik B, Klingberg G. Dental treatment, dental fear and behavior management problems in children with severe enamel hypomineralization of their permanent molars. Int J Paediatr Dent. 2002;12(1):24–32.
2. William V, Burrow M, Palamara J, Messer L. Microshear bond strength of resin composite to teeth affected by molar incisor hypomineralization using 2 adhesive systems. Pediatr Dent. 2006;28(3):233–41.
3. Lygidakis N. Treatment modalities in children with teeth affected by molar-incisor enamel hypomineralisation (MIH): a systematic review. Eur Arch Paediatr Dent. 2010;11(2):65–74.
4. American Academy of Pediatric Dentistry. Guideline on pulp therapy for primary and immature permanent teeth. Pediatr Dent. 2010;35(6):235–42.
5. Zagdwon A, Fayle S, Pollard M. A prospective clinical trial comparing preformed metal crowns and cast restorations for defective first permanent molars. Eur J Paediatr Dent. 2003;4(3):138–42.
6. Sandler P, Atkinson R, Murray A. For four sixes. Am J Orthod Dentofacial Orthop. 2000;117(4):418–34.
7. Koch M, Garcia-Godoy F. The clinical performance of laboratory-fabricated crowns placed on first permanent molars with developmental defects. J Am Dent Assoc. 2000;131(9):1285–90.
8. Jälevik B, Moller M. Evaluation of spontaneous space closure and development of permanent dentition after extraction of hypomineralized permanent first molars. Int J Paediatr Dent. 2007;17(5):328–35.
9. Mejare I, Bergman E, Grindefjord M. Hypomineralized molars and incisors of unknown origin: treatment outcome at age 18 years. Int J Paediatr Dent. 2005;15(1):20–8.
10. Teo T, Ashley P, Parekh S. The evaluation of spontaneous space closure after the extraction of first permanent molars. Eur Arch Paediatr Dent. 2013;14(4):207–12.
11. Williams R, Hosila L. The effects of different extraction sites upon incisor retraction. Am J Orthod. 1976;69(4):388–410.
12. Gill D, Lee R, Tredwin C. Treatment planning for the loss of first permanent molars. Dent Updat. 2001;28:304–8.
13. Ong D-V, Bleakley J. Compromised first permanent molars: an orthodontic perspective. Aust Dent J. 2010;55(1):2–14.
14. Yavuz I, Baydas B, Ikbal A, Daǧsuyu M, Ceylan I. Effects of early loss of permanent first molars on the development of third molars. Am J Orthod Dentofacial Orthop. 2006;130(5):634–8.
15. Çaǧlaroǧlu M, Kilic N, Erdem A. Effects of early unilateral first molar extraction on skeletal asymmetry. Am J Orthod Dentofacial Orthop. 2008;134(2):270–5.

16. Richardson A. Spontaneous changes in the incisor relationship following extraction of lower first permanent molars. Br J Orthod. 1979;6(2):85–90.
17. Cobourne M, Williams A, McMullen R. A guideline for the extraction of first permanent molars in children. London: Royal College of Surgeons of England; 2009.
18. Thunold K. Early loss of the first molars 25 years later. Rep Congr Eur Orthod Soc. 1970:349–65.

Managing the Prevention of Dental Caries and Sensitivity in Teeth with Enamel Defects

9

Felicity Crombie and David J. Manton

Abstract

Developmental defects of enamel (DDE) may affect either or both the quality and the quantity of enamel and as such potentially have implications for caries risk and hypersensitivity. The management of these teeth in terms of caries prevention/tooth structure preservation and sensitivity often overlaps and so is presented together. This chapter proposes strategies to address the fundamental deficiencies of the enamel and to optimize clinical and patient outcomes. Earliest possible intervention is advocated and includes oral hygiene, diet and salivary advice, mineralization therapy, and surface sealants. These are all broadly familiar to the clinician from the caries context, but some modifications are recommended when applied to developmental defects. Less familiar techniques, such as the potential applications for recently developed infiltrant resin materials, as well as full coverage "sealants" for severely affected teeth, are also presented.

Introduction

When considering dental caries and sensitivity, the clinician should understand that enamel defects, either developmental or acquired, fall within one or both of two categories: defects of enamel *quantity* and/or defects of enamel *quality*. The relative caries or posteruptive breakdown (PEB) risk, mechanism of hypersensitivity, and therefore appropriate management are to a large extent determined by the type of defect. Hypersensitivity tends to be associated more with hypomineralized enamel

F. Crombie, BDSc (Hons), PhD
Growth and Development Unit, Melbourne Dental School, University of Melbourne, Melbourne, VIC 3010, Australia
e-mail: fcrombie@unimelb.edu.au

D.J. Manton, BDSc, MDSc, PhD (✉)
Growth and Development Unit, Melbourne Dental School, University of Melbourne, 720 Swanston St, Carlton, VIC 3053, Australia
e-mail: djmanton@unimelb.edu.au

© Springer-Verlag Berlin Heidelberg 2015
B.K. Drummond, N. Kilpatrick (eds.), *Planning and Care for Children and Adolescents with Dental Enamel Defects: Etiology, Research and Contemporary Management*, DOI 10.1007/978-3-662-44800-7_9

than with hypoplastic enamel; however, each individual should be managed in a manner appropriate to their particular presenting problems.

The enamel should be the hardest tissue in the human body and, if healthy, allows the teeth to withstand normal functional loading. The enamel protects the underlying dentine and therefore limits the relatively more rapid progression of caries and wear in dentine compared to enamel – this protection or lack of it can also moderate dentinal sensitivity. In order to fulfill these demands, enamel is a highly specialized and organized tissue and aberrations often result in catastrophic reductions in performance, as discussed in Chap. 6. The underlying mechanisms leading to hypersensitivity are probably linked to reduced enamel thickness in the case of hypoplasia and increased porosity in severely hypomineralized enamel. Generally (but not always) the hypersensitivity, particularly in hypomineralized enamel, occurs following PEB and in some cases is exacerbated by an underlying pulpitis [1]. Many of the properties and processes contributing to hypersensitivity are also implicated in caries risk, and so management strategies often overlap. Management can be complicated by the age and compliance of the patient [2, 3].

Dental Caries and Erosion Risk

Research has established that enamel surface integrity and bacterial adhesion are important in caries initiation. While it has been well documented in the primary dentition that the relatively reduced thickness and poorer structure of enamel can be linked to an increased rate of caries progression [4, 5], the evidence in the permanent dentition is equivocal. Enamel defects are often vulnerable from both perspectives with hypoplasia or PEB not only reducing the thickness of the protective enamel layer but potentially creating non-cleansable contours. Furthermore in hypomineralized defects apparently intact surfaces frequently display surface irregularities and porosities on a microscopic scale (Fig. 9.1 – SEM image of pitted enamel surface). The susceptibility of these qualitative defects to dental caries can be compounded by increased porosity and in some cases, such as in molar incisor hypomineralization (MIH) and hypocalcification/hypomaturation types of amelogenesis imperfecta (AI), decreased mineral and increased protein content, and decreased hardness and increased solubility of enamel [6–8]. The management of

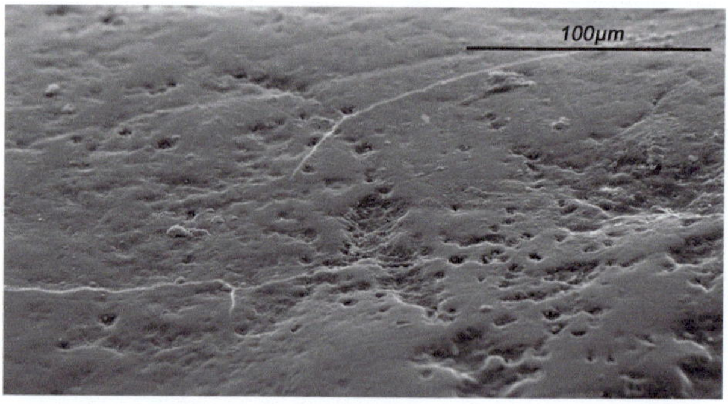

Fig. 9.1 Surface of a clinically intact MIH lesion viewed under a scanning electron microscope showing characteristic surface irregularities (×1000 mag)

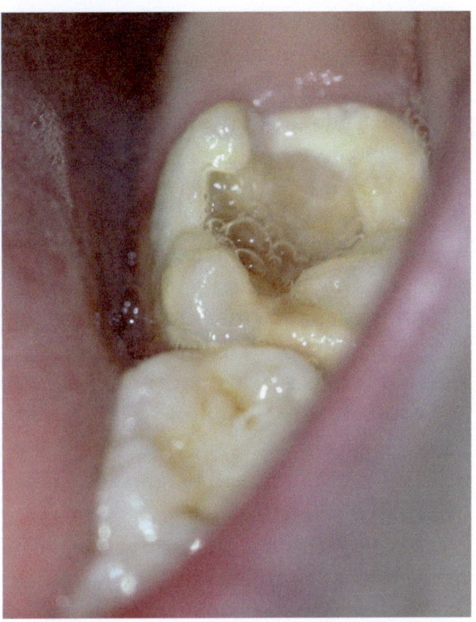

Fig. 9.2 MIH-affected tooth with severe loss of structure and caries before complete eruption

hypoplastic, quantitative defects usually focuses on establishing a cleansable surface, with the use of materials such as flowable resin composite to replace deficient enamel and create a smooth and cleansable surface. However, more extensive restorative care such as full coverage restorations may be required if the hypoplastic defects are severe [2]. It should be noted that in the case of enamel defects, establishing cleansable surfaces is not purely related to contour and may also require control of sensitivity to allow adequate oral hygiene to be performed [2, 3].

For qualitative defects, improving physical and chemical properties to optimize preservation and improvement of hypomineralized enamel tissue is the primary goal. Most strategies utilized clinically for hypomineralized enamel defects are based on the standard caries disease model, such as minimization of caries risk. However, some of these cannot always be applied directly to developmentally defective tissues because of the defective structure [2, 9]. Most particularly, in severe hypomineralization cases, intervention must be instituted as early as possible since significant damage can occur even before the crown is fully erupted (see Fig. 9.2). Anterior teeth are less affected by PEB and are less likely to become carious after enamel loss. However, molar teeth with PEB are at risk and should be closely monitored [10].

Prevention of Dental Caries and Erosion

To achieve success with any preventive strategy, early and accurate diagnosis is critical (see Chaps. 1, 2, 3, and 5). Once a diagnosis has been made, it is essential to emphasize the importance of general preventive principles for these teeth and to recognize that otherwise acceptable levels of care and compliance may be insufficient for caries prevention in these more vulnerable teeth. Where clinicians note that primary second molars or permanent incisors have DDE, this indicates the first permanent molars may also be affected and consideration should be given to altering recall timing and/or frequency to facilitate earliest possible intervention [11, 12]. If the case appears to be severe or complex, especially for genetic conditions such as AI or where sedation or general anesthesia may be required, early specialist referral to plan longer-term interventions may be the most appropriate management a general practitioner can provide (Chaps. 10 and 11).

Oral hygiene instruction should be undertaken including advice to ensure partially erupted teeth are cleaned appropriately – often using a buccolingual stroke with a soft brush for partially erupted molars to improve efficacy of plaque removal during the long eruption phase [13]. Given defects often manifest at an early age, before independent oral hygiene is recommended, the use of disclosing agents can assist both children and parents to better visualize deposits on the teeth. For sensitive teeth the simple suggestion to use warm water with the toothpaste when brushing may be helpful. Defects affecting the primary dentition may encourage increased cariogenic bacteria colonization with consequent higher caries risk. Although this has not been a consistent finding, it may still be prudent to include advice to reduce caries risk even when there has been little past evidence of caries [14, 15].

Dietary counseling, ideally in the form of a motivational interview where by providing information in a collaborative manner, encouraging willingness, ability, and readiness the clinician facilitates rather than directs change [16], is recommended [17]. This may include advice on caries prevention as well as on managing hypersensitivity, which is often as simple as avoiding or decreasing causative factors – i.e., cold drinks or food. As with standard dietary counseling, the role of fermentable carbohydrates (especially sucrose), particularly in terms of frequency and duration, should be discussed along with strategies to minimize exposures and ideas for healthier alternatives [18]. Intrinsic and/or extrinsic acids may also warrant some discussion not only in terms of exacerbating sensitivity but also, particularly in generalized conditions such as AI, because they may accelerate enamel loss in the form of erosive tooth wear. The influence of salivary characteristics should also be considered and potentially integrated into dietary counseling. As there is some evidence to suggest that salivary protection is less favorable in children affected by MIH, testing of salivary characteristics such as flow and consistency may be of benefit [14].

Preventive Agents

Another core component of caries prevention and desensitization is the use of fluoridated agents and calcium-based remineralizing agents. Ideally, for qualitative defects, the aim is not merely to remineralize any posteruptive demineralization but to address the primary mineral deficiency [19]. Studies of MIH, both in vivo and in vitro, suggest that casein phosphopeptide-amorphous calcium phosphate with

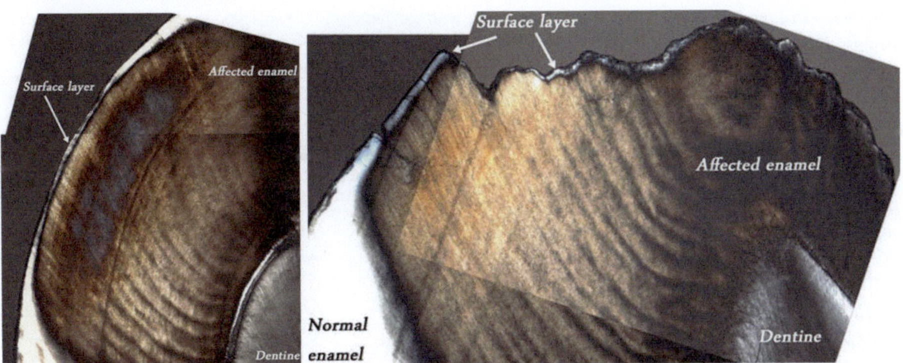

Fig. 9.3 Polarized light images of surface layer observed on both intact and PEB surfaces of MIH-affected teeth (in water, ×5 mag.). *White/gray* indicates reduced porosity (≤5 %), *brown/orange* indicates increased porosity (>5 %)

and without fluoride (CPP-ACFP/ACP) application can improve enamel mineral content and reduce porosity both on exposed surfaces and deeper within the enamel tissue (see Fig. 9.3) [19, 20]. It is believed that a smoother surface, denser structure, and additional mineral content, especially if it is in the more chemically favorable forms of fluorapatite or fluoridated hydroxyapatite, should putatively reduce caries and breakdown risk [19].

The action of CPP-based products relates to the ability of this milk-based protein to stabilize calcium and phosphate in high concentration and provide supersaturated ionic calcium and phosphate at and below the tooth surface. This then allows the diffusion of calcium and phosphate ions down a concentration gradient into the lesion at much higher concentrations than otherwise would be possible driving remineralization [21]. Reducing porosity is also likely to translate into a reduction in clinical sensitivity. Most reports of improvement in hypersensitivity are anecdotal; however, fluoride and remineralization treatments are consistently recommended in the literature, although a strong evidence base is lacking. There may be some additional benefit gained by prior deproteinization treatment; a similar finding has been reported for fluorosed enamel [19, 22]. In both of these cases, this was achieved by irrigation with a sodium hypochlorite solution (NaOCl); however, the clinical applicability/practicalities need to be considered given the likely difficulties in achieving adequate isolation and comfort. When NaOCl is used, the tooth needs to be completely isolated by sealed rubber dam, and as these teeth are often partially erupted, this may be difficult to achieve as may be adequate local analgesia. The leakage of the NaOCl into the oral cavity would have significant consequences.

Children with significant hypersensitivity or deemed at higher caries risk should be prescribed an optimal-strength fluoride toothpaste under appropriate professional and parental supervision. Anecdotally, frequent use of stannous fluoride has appeared to improve sensitivity in hypomineralized teeth; however, evidence is lacking. For very young children where controlling fluoride ingestion may be difficult, a calcium phosphate-based product would be recommended initially in

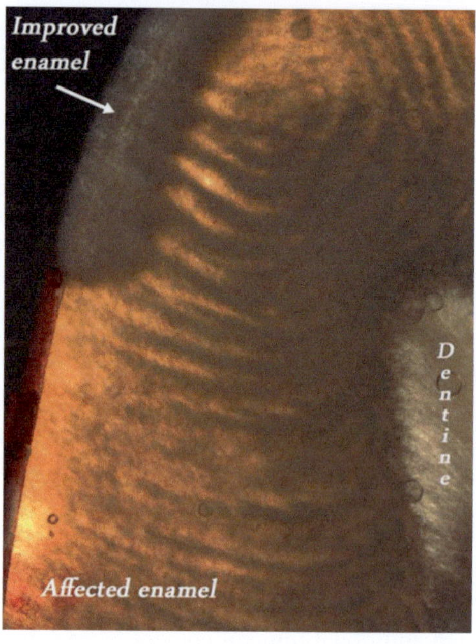

Fig. 9.4 Polarized light image of an MIH lesion following exposure to a CPP-ACFP solution in vitro (in water, ×5 mag.). *Brown/orange* area is the unchanged lesion (>5 % porosity), *gray* area (5 % porosity) shows the part of the lesion exposed to the solution, while the red surface coating protects the unexposed (control) part of the lesion

conjunction with professional application of a fluoride varnish or a stannous fluoride gel. It seems likely that the greatest gains of continuing mineralization will be made as the teeth emerge. Like demineralization lesions, hypomineralized enamel defects have been shown to develop a thin but relatively well-mineralized surface layer which helps prevent further loss of minerals but can inhibit subsequent, deeper tissue improvement in mineral content (see Fig. 9.4) [6].

Surface Sealing

Sealants

In more severe hypomineralization cases, preventive measures alone are often insufficient and some form of surface protection is indicated [23]. At its simplest this will be standard sealing and this is recommended prior to full emergence of the tooth [24]. A glass ionomer cement (GIC) material is therefore the best initial choice as it can tolerate the presence of some moisture and can provide a source of ions which appear to be advantageous to the underlying tooth in several ways. An incidental finding of an MIH characterization study suggested that deeper mineralization improvements occur under a GIC sealant compared with enamel surfaces exposed to the oral environment [25]. It has been reported that GIC materials also provide a "halo protection" effect, whereby healthy enamel immediately adjacent to a GIC material is less susceptible to demineralization, which may be further enhanced by the addition of CPP-ACP to the GIC [26]. Where PEB has already occurred, protective sealing may be extended over all the affected areas to decrease caries risk until such time that more definitive treatment can be undertaken. Where sealing cannot be achieved, full coverage options should be considered (Chaps. 10 and 11). Once isolation can be established, there are more clinical options available (Chap. 11). However, resin-based sealants are not always recommended because of the difficulties in bonding to enamel that is hypomineralized and has a higher protein content (see Chap. 6). It is widely reported that enamel defects display atypical and often poor etch patterns (Chap. 6) with implications for bonding of resin materials including resin sealants [27–30]. Extended etching times for severely fluorotic enamel are recommended because of the increased resistance of fluorapatite to acidic dissolution [27]. There is some evidence to suggest that the higher organic content of defective enamel limits remineralization and reduces bond strengths. Techniques such as irrigation with NaOCl can remove protein and improve bonding and penetration of resin materials in MIH and AI [29, 31–33]. It appears important that to increase bond strengths, the NaOCl should be used after etching, not before [29, 34, 35].

Methods reported to increase bond strengths and retention rates of resin-based sealants to intact hypomineralized occlusal surfaces have involved the use of a single-bottle adhesive system (One-Step®, Bisco, IL, USA) and pretreatment with NaOCl after etching. Resin infiltration with materials such as Icon (DMG, Hamburg, Germany) has been reported to increase bond strengths in vitro; however, whether this decreases sensitivity and PEB is unknown [29, 34, 36].

Resin Infiltration

The recent development of a commercial resin infiltrant for treatment of carious lesions has led to some preliminary studies to see if this low-viscosity TEGMA resin can be used to seal and improve the physical qualities of hypomineralized enamel. There is little published research; however, what exists indicates that while the pattern of infiltration is hard to predict, it is possible to obtain resin penetration close to the amelodentinal junction (ADJ) [36, 37]. Where infiltration was achieved there was an increase in cross-sectional hardness of the enamel [36]. The effect of pretreatment with NaOCl improved infiltration. However, further research is required before this can be recommended as routine treatment [36]. There has also been some initial *in vitro* research suggesting that the use of NaOCl after etching, followed by a resin infiltrant prior to bonding, may increase bond strengths. The pros and cons of the clinical applicability of this increased complexity and cost need to be investigated and discussed.

Other Sealing Methods

In some children and adolescents, full coverage of affected teeth may be required in a protective rather than reparative capacity [3]. This may be for two reasons – protection of friable structure and decreasing sensitivity. In the case of a generalized defect such as AI, composite strip crowns on anterior teeth and preformed metal crowns on posterior teeth (cemented with GIC) may be appropriate. This can be definitive for the primary dentition and transitional for the permanent dentition (Chaps. 10 and 11).

There has been some suggestion for the use of a technique modified after that of Zagdwon et al. where preformed crowns are placed over severely hypomineralized permanent molars with as little tooth preparation as possible [38]. This technique often involves the of use orthodontic separators to create space for the crown, reducing the need for interproximal preparation. The minimal occlusal preparation does cause an increase in vertical dimension. However, in children this spontaneously decreases over the course of a couple of months. The pulpal status of the tooth needs to be at a stage where any inflammatory changes present are reversible. This technique is similar to the "Hall technique" advocated recently for the treatment of initial lesions in primary teeth which relies on the sealing of the lesion from the oral environment, thereby stopping progression of any caries and also protecting developmental weakened tooth structure [39]. While results for the Hall technique are promising, further research is required in this area, particularly in the context of developmental defects.

Summary

For hypoplastic defects, the provision of a cleansable surface is the most effective way of decreasing caries risk – this may be achieved with resin composites or full coverage. Sensitivity is less of an issue with these teeth, but if it is present, similar techniques to those for hypomineralization defects are appropriate.

For hypomineralized defects, maintenance of the enamel surface integrity and limitation of sensitivity are essential. Increase in caries risk due to the inability to clean the hypomineralized area can lead to PEB. Therefore the conditions should be seen as interrelated. Adherence to the modified recommendations according to William et al. [40] and Oliver et al. [10] is appropriate (see Table 9.1).

Table 9.1 Clinical management tree for hypomineralized teeth

Steps	Procedures
Hypomineralization risk identification	Assess medical history for putative etiological factors
	Establish caries risk and modify as necessary
Early diagnosis	Examine at-risk molars as they erupt especially if permanent incisors, second primary molars, or other teeth are affected. Assess severity
Remineralization	Apply topical fluoride and calcium-based products such as CPP-ACP. Consider "adult strength" toothpaste. Minimize caries risk
Desensitization	Assess for remineralization. Protect porous lesions with GIC or resin sealant. Decrease exposure to acidic drinks
Prevention of caries and PEB	Assess for remineralization and desensitization. Consider full coverage of tooth if at high potential for PEB

References

1. Rodd HD, Boissonade FP, Day PF. Pulpal status of hypomineralized permanent molars. Pediatr Dent. 2007;29(6):514–20.
2. McDonald S, Arkutu N, Malik K, Gadhia K, McKaig S. Managing the paediatric patient with amelogenesis imperfecta. Br Dent J. 2012;212(9):425–8.
3. Weerheijm KL. Molar Incisor Hypomineralization (MIH): clinical presentation, aetiology and management. Dent Updat. 2004;31(1):9–12.
4. Wang LJ, Tang R, Bonstein T, Bush P, Nancollas GH. Enamel demineralization in primary and permanent teeth. J Dent Res. 2006;85(4):359–63.
5. Salanitri S, Seow WK. Developmental enamel defects in the primary dentition: aetiology and clinical management. Aust Dent J. 2013;58(2):133–40.
6. Crombie F, Manton D, Palamara J, Zalizniak I, Cochrane N, Reynolds E. Characterisation of developmentally hypomineralised human enamel. J Dent. 2013;41(7):611–8.
7. Wright JT. Amelogenesis imperfecta. Eur J Oral Sci. 2011;119 Suppl 1:338–41.
8. Elfrink MEC, ten Cate JM, van Ruijven LJ, Veerkamp JSJ. Mineral content in teeth with Deciduous Molar Hypomineralisation (DMH). J Dent. 2013;41(11):974–8.
9. Featherstone JDB. Remineralization, the natural caries repair process – the need for new approaches. Adv Dent Res. 2009;21(1):4–7.
10. Oliver K, Messer LB, Manton DJ, Kan K, Ng F, Olsen CB, et al. Distribution and severity of molar hypomineralisation: trial of a new severity index. Int J Paediatr Dent. 2013;24(2):131–51.
11. Elfrink MEC, ten Cate JM, Jaddoe VWV, Hofman A, Moll HA, Veerkamp JSJ. Deciduous molar hypomineralization and molar incisor hypomineralization. J Dent Res. 2012;91(6): 551–5.
12. Ghanim A, Manton D, Marino R, Morgan M, Bailey D. Prevalence of demarcated hypomineralisation defects in second primary molars in Iraqi children. Int J Paediatr Dent. 2013;23(1):48–55.
13. Frazão P. Effectiveness of the bucco-lingual technique within a school-based supervised toothbrushing program on preventing caries: a randomized controlled trial. BMC Oral Health. 2011;11(1):11.
14. Ghanim A, Marino R, Morgan M, Bailey D, Manton D. An in vivo investigation of salivary properties, enamel hypomineralisation, and carious lesion severity in a group of Iraqi schoolchildren. Int J Paediatr Dent. 2013;23(1):2–12.
15. Hong L, Levy SM, Warren JJ, Broffitt B. Association between enamel hypoplasia and dental caries in primary second molars: a cohort study. Caries Res. 2009;43(5):345–53.
16. Martins RK, McNeil DW. Review of motivational interviewing in promoting health behaviors. Clin Psychol Rev. 2009;29(4):283–93.
17. Harrison R, Benton T, Everson-Stewart S, Weinstein P. Effect of motivational interviewing on rates of early childhood caries: a randomized trial. Pediatr Dent. 2007;29(1):16–22.
18. Moynihan PJ, Kelly SAM. Effect on caries of restricting sugars intake: systematic review to inform WHO guidelines. J Dent Res. 2014;93(1):8–18.
19. Crombie F, Cochrane N, Manton D, Palamara J, Reynolds E. Mineralisation of developmentally hypomineralised human enamel in vitro. Caries Res. 2013;47(3):259–63.
20. Baroni C, Marchionni S. MIH supplementation strategies prospective clinical and laboratory trial. J Dent Res. 2011;90(3):371–6.
21. Cochrane N, Cai F, Huq N, Burrow M, Reynolds E. New approaches to enhanced remineralization of tooth enamel. J Dent Res. 2010;89(11):1187–97.
22. Den Besten P, Giambro N. Treatment of fluorosed and white-spot human enamel with calcium sucrose phosphate in vitro. Pediatr Dent. 1995;17:340–5.
23. Wright JT. The etch-bleach-seal technique for managing stained enamel defects in young permanent incisors. Pediatr Dent. 2002;24:249–52.
24. Lygidakis NA, Wong F, Jälevik B, Vierrou AM, Alaluusua S, Espelid I. Best clinical practice guidance for clinicians dealing with children presenting with Molar-Incisor-Hypomineralisation (MIH). Eur Arch Paediatr Dent. 2010;11(2):75–81.

25. Crombie F, Manton D, Reynolds E. Therapie der Molaren-Inzisiven-Hypomineralisation (MIH) in einem schwierigen Umfeld" (German translation of MIH – Therapy with difficult conditions, special characteristics of MIH teeth). Quintessenz. 2011;62(12):1593–9.

26. Zalizniak I, Palamara J, Wong R, Cochrane N, Burrow M, Reynolds E. Ion release and physical properties of CPP-ACP modified GIC in acid solutions. J Dent. 2013;41(5):449–54.

27. Al-Sugair M, Akpata E. Effect of fluorosis on etching of human enamel. J Oral Rehab. 1999;26(6):521–8.

28. William V, Burrow MF, Palamara JE, Messer LB. Microshear bond strength of resin composite to teeth affected by molar hypomineralization using 2 adhesive systems. Pediatr Dent. 2006;28(3):233–41.

29. Chay P, Manton D, Palamara J. The effect of resin infiltration and oxidative pre-treatment on microshear bond strength of resin composite to hypomineralised enamel. Int J Paediatr Dent. 2014;24(4):252–67.

30. Torres-Gallegos I, Zavala-Alonso V, Patiño-Marín N, Martinez-Castañon G, Anusavice K, Loyola-Rodríguez J. Enamel roughness and depth profile after phosphoric acid etching of healthy and fluorotic enamel. Aust Dent J. 2012;57(2):151–6.

31. Farah RA, Monk BC, Swain MV, Drummond BK. Protein content of molar–incisor hypomineralisation enamel. J Dent. 2010;38(7):591–6.

32. Mangum JE, Crombie FA, Kilpatrick N, Manton DJ, Hubbard MJ. Surface integrity governs the proteome of hypomineralized enamel. J Dent Res. 2010;89(10):1160–5.

33. Venezie RD, Vadiakas G, Christensen JR, Wright J. Enamel pretreatment with sodium hypochlorite to enhance bonding in hypocalcified amelogenesis imperfecta: case report and SEM analysis. Pediatr Dent. 1994;16:433–6.

34. Şaroğlu I, Aras Ş, Öztaş D. Effect of deproteinization on composite bond strength in hypocalcified amelogenesis imperfecta. Oral Dis. 2006;12(3):305–8.

35. Gandhi S, Crawford P, Shellis P. The use of a 'bleach-etch-seal'deproteinization technique on MIH affected enamel. Int J Paediatr Dent. 2012;22(6):427–34.

36. Crombie F, Manton D, Palamara J, Reynolds E. Resin infiltration of developmentally hypomineralised enamel. Int J Paediatr Dent. 2014;24(1):51–5.

37. Natarajan AK. Characterisation of enamel and effect of resin infiltration in molar-incisor hypomineralisation. University of Otago. Thesis, Doctor of Clinical Dentistry; 2013. Retrieved from http://hdl.handle.net/10523/4471 on 10 Mar 2014.

38. Zagdwon AM, Fayle SA, Pollard MA. A prospective clinical trial comparing preformed metal crowns and cast restorations for defective first permanent molars. Eur J Paediatr Dent. 2003;4(3):138–42.

39. Ricketts D, Kidd E, Innes N, Clarkson J. Complete or ultraconservative removal of decayed tissue in unfilled teeth. Cochrane Database Syst Rev. 2006;3, CD003808.

40. William V, Messer L, Burrow M. Molar incisor hypomineralization: review and recommendations for clinical management. Pediatr Dent. 2006;28(3):224–32.

Restorative Management of Dental Enamel Defects in the Primary Dentition

10

Monty Duggal and Hani Nazzal

Abstract

Many genetic and environmental conditions can interfere with the normal development of primary teeth and can manifest as defects in the enamel. Such defects can be associated with pain and discomfort and can have esthetic implications which may affect the young child's self-esteem. It is not only important for clinicians to be able to diagnose the defects but also to understand the implications these might have on restorative techniques and materials they choose. Restorative management can be challenging because of the limited cooperation in some children, the extent of the defects, and the sensitivity that may be present. The main aims of treatment should be to alleviate pain and sensitivity, improve esthetics, and manage any other concerns that the child or the parents might have. This should be followed by consideration of long-term treatment planning involving progression of the primary through to the mixed dentition. In many cases, especially where there is a genetic component with generalized involvement of both the primary and subsequent permanent teeth, an interdisciplinary approach to management is appropriate. Finally it is important to be able to provide treatment in a manner the child finds acceptable. This chapter helps the reader identify and effectively manage primary teeth with commonly encountered enamel defects.

M. Duggal, BDS, MDSc, PhD
Department of Paediatric Dentistry, School of Dentistry, University of Leeds,
Clarendon Way, Leeds, West Yorkshire LS29LU, UK
e-mail: m.s.duggal@leeds.ac.uk

H. Nazzal, BDS, PhD (✉)
Department of Paediatric Dentistry, School of Dentistry, University of Leeds,
Clarendon Way, Leeds, West Yorkshire WF1 4JN, UK
e-mail: denha@leeds.ac.uk

© Springer-Verlag Berlin Heidelberg 2015

123

B.K. Drummond, N. Kilpatrick (eds.), *Planning and Care for Children and Adolescents with Dental Enamel Defects: Etiology, Research and Contemporary Management*, DOI 10.1007/978-3-662-44800-7_10

Introduction

In this chapter the management of developmental defects of enamel (DDE) in children is discussed, and the choice of techniques and materials, which are appropriate in the growing child, is elaborated upon. An important consideration is that many affected children will not have had any invasive dental treatment before. Suggested strategies for managing young children are included.

Etiology of DDE in the Primary Dentition

The etiology of DDE in the primary dentition can be divided into systemic and local causes. Local factors affecting primary teeth are limited to traumatic injuries. This is occasionally seen following neonatal intubation or the use of an oral airway for an extended period of time [1]. However, this has to occur at a very young age, i.e., before birth or during infancy, for it to affect enamel formation of the anterior primary teeth, making this an unusual phenomenon. Systemic factors, on the other hand, are more common and comprise a variety of conditions [2, 3] which are summarized in Table 10.1 below and discussed in more detail in Chaps. 1, 2, 3, and 4.

Unlike genetically determined defects, the effect of developmental factors on enamel formation depends upon the timing, duration, and severity of these factors and is usually referred to as chronological hypoplasia/hypomineralization (Fig. 10.1). For these factors to affect the formation of enamel in primary teeth, they will occur during hard tissue formation of the primary teeth. This starts with central incisor formation at 13–16 weeks after fertilization and ends with the second primary molars at 8–11 months of age [4]. The type of resulting defect will reflect whether the insult occurred during enamel matrix formation (leading to hypoplasia), mineralization (causing hypocalcification defects), or during maturation phase (causing hypomaturation defects). A clinician is likely to encounter two main types of enamel defects: hypoplastic and hypomineralized enamel. Hypoplastic enamel [4, 5] (Fig. 10.2) is caused by incomplete or defective formation of the organic

Table 10.1 Systemic factors that may be associated with DDE in primary teeth

Factors	Examples
Genetically determined	Amelogenesis imperfecta [3]
Chromosomal anomalies	Down syndrome
Congenital defects	Cardiac defects, unilateral facial hypoplasia or hypertrophy [2]
Inborn errors of metabolism	Galactosemia, phenylketonuria, alkaptonuria, erythropoietic porphyria, primary hyperoxaluria
Neonatal disturbances	Prematurity, hypokalemia
Infectious diseases	Measles, chickenpox
Neurological disturbances	
Chronic medical diseases	Hepatic disease, endocrinopathies, renal disease, enteropathies
Maternal health during pregnancy	Hypertension, nutritional deficiency, substance abuse
Nutritional deficiencies	Vit. D deficiency

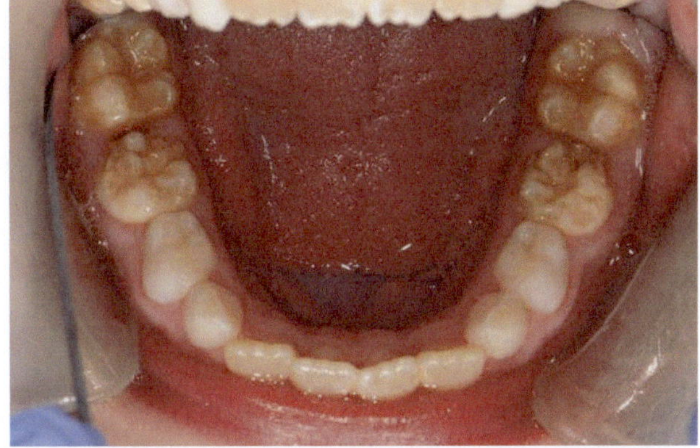

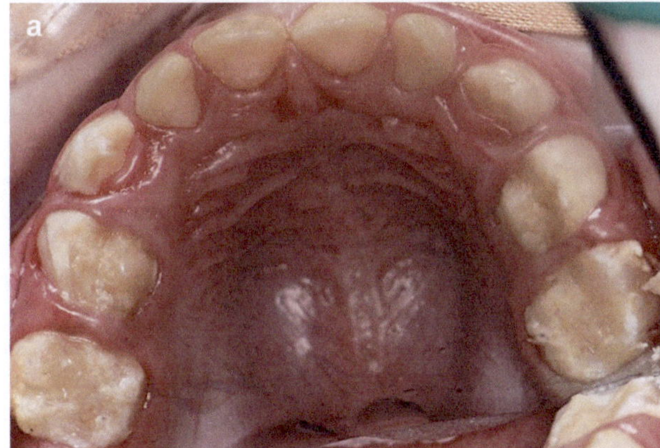

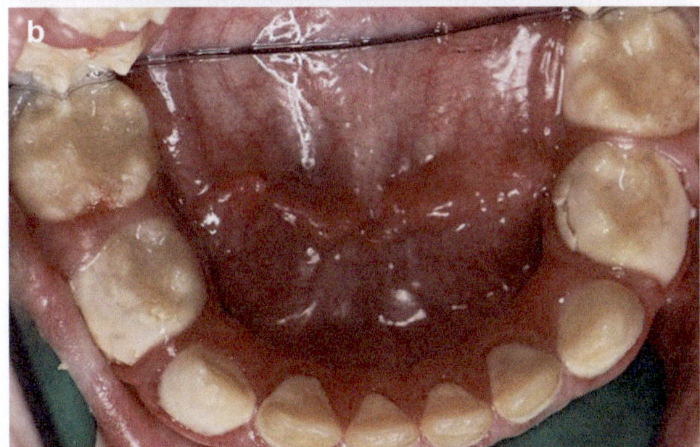

Fig. 10.1 Chronological hypoplasia affecting the lower second primary molars and chronological hypomineralization affecting lower first permanent molars

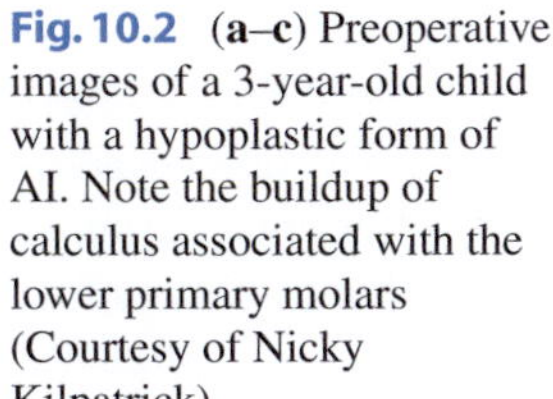

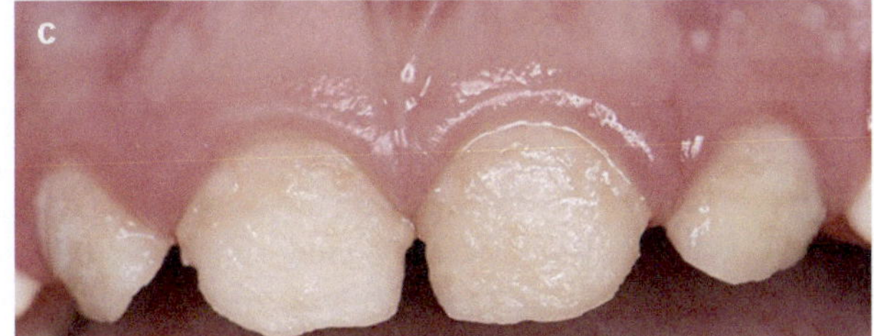

Fig. 10.2 (**a–c**) Preoperative images of a 3-year-old child with a hypoplastic form of AI. Note the buildup of calculus associated with the lower primary molars (Courtesy of Nicky Kilpatrick)

enamel matrix by ameloblasts during tooth formation (secretory stage) resulting in thinner but normally mineralized enamel. Hypomineralization occurs due to a failure in enamel matrix mineralization [4, 5]. This is further divided into hypocalcification (defective mineralization) or hypomaturation (defective removal of proteins from enamel matrix preventing maturation). Clinically, hypocalcified enamel is usually yellow-brown in color with more potential for enamel breakdown, while hypomature enamel may appear normal, mottled, or slightly opaque [4, 5].

Management of DDE in Primary Teeth

The management of enamel defects in generalized conditions or where they are likely to affect the permanent dentition is challenging and usually requires immediate-, short- and long-term planning [6]. Patients with amelogenesis imperfecta (AI), for instance, may have other associated anomalies such as disturbances in eruption, anterior open bite, pulpal calcifications, pathological root or crown resorption, and/or taurodontism. These anomalies affect the long-term management and usually require an interdisciplinary approach starting in the later primary/early mixed dentition. Patients with primary teeth defects often present at a young age and the parents want immediate treatment to improve the child's appearance. However, it is important to make a treatment plan which will encompass a stepwise approach that includes a short-, medium-, and a long-term treatment plan. Children with DDE often require several interventions throughout their primary, mixed, and permanent dentition stages [7], and should general anesthesia (GA) be required, it is crucial to plan and provide the necessary management in a timely manner so that the least number of GAs are required throughout the child's life.

The aims of management, especially at the primary dentition stage, include:

1. Prevention and maintenance of good oral hygiene
2. Desensitization and pain management of affected teeth
3. Restorative management (esthetic management and stabilization of affected teeth)
4. Behavior management to help children manage the dental care they need

Prevention

The gingival condition and oral hygiene of patients with both generalized defects, such as in AI or isolated defects, are often poor. Figures 10.1 and 10.3 show the presence of calculus in children with hypoplastic and hypomineralized AI. This occurs because many of the teeth are sensitive to thermal and toothbrush stimuli, which prohibits effective toothbrushing. Having enamel defects can also be an additional caries risk factor as the teeth are rough and porous with softer and/or thinner enamel. Therefore, treatment planning should firstly focus on prevention including effective oral hygiene instruction using warm water and very soft brushes,

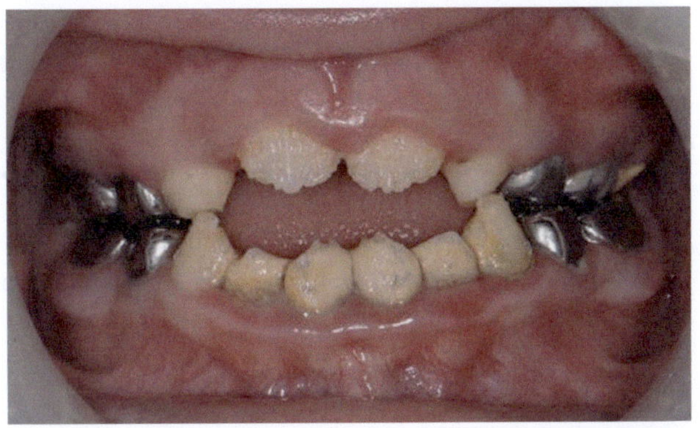

Fig. 10.3 Anterior view of the mixed dentition in a child with AI showing poor oral hygiene, calculus deposits, and gingivitis

optimizing fluoride exposure both at home and with regular professional application, diet advice and sealants, or temporary restorations where appropriate. A guide is given in the UK Department of Health and British Association for the Study of Community Dentistry toolkit [8]. Comprehensive dietary analysis and advice is essential from both a caries and tooth surface-loss perspective. This will involve identifying fermentable carbohydrates and acidic foods and beverages in the diet and advising on their reduction and timing of use to minimize damage.

It is unrealistic to expect children with DDE to dramatically improve their oral hygiene without some intervention to reduce the sensitivity of the teeth. This might include the use of preventive agents such as topical fluorides or calcium phosphate-containing products or by placing interim restorations (glass ionomer cements or compomers) that will seal the dentine, thereby allowing the child to brush the affected teeth with less discomfort. In younger children, below 6 years-of-age, parents should help with brushing twice daily and should carry out regular flossing if the contact areas are closed.

Reducing Sensitivity

Several strategies are available for the treatment of the sensitivity associated with DDE, although none have been found to be reliable for every case (see Chap. 9). It is important to consider desensitization in order to reduce the discomfort felt by many children with DDE. This sensitivity also makes restorative interventions, especially with adhesive materials, even more challenging. Some of the suggested methods for desensitization include the use of topical fluoride preparations, in particular fluoride varnishes, such as Duraphat® 22,600 ppm F (Colgate Oral Care) or 3M Espe Fluoride Varnish with tricalcium phosphate. Care should be taken to use the recommended amounts on erupting teeth with DDE in preschool-aged children. More recently a combination of casein phosphopeptide and amorphous calcium phosphate (CPP-ACP – GC Tooth Mousse/MI Paste) with and without fluoride has also been advocated to help decrease sensitivity. CPP-ACP helps create, stabilize, and deposit a supersaturated solution of calcium and phosphate at the enamel surface. Therefore, it has been suggested that home application of a CPP-ACP-containing cream especially when combined with fluoride use will help remineralize and desensitize by acting as a source of bioavailable calcium and phosphate. Other topical fluorides may also be useful; among these are stannous fluoride gels, such as Gel-Kam® 1,000 ppm F (Colgate Oral Care) or OMNI Gel 0.4 %/1,000 ppm F (3M). There has also been a suggestion that desensitizing toothpastes may help with some hypomineralized teeth. Currently there is no strong evidence to support the efficacy of these strategies in the management of DDE, though all these products may help reduce sensitivity and enhance mineralization of the hypomineralized areas. However, none of the available products are always effective, and clinicians should consider using products in combination or trying different products in an attempt to alleviate the symptoms in patients.

Pain and Anxiety Management

Pain management in children is an integral part of good pediatric dentistry. Both the technique and choice of local analgesia are important for the provision of high quality, effective restorations in children, particularly if they are to last for the lifetime of the primary teeth (up to 8 years). In particular, teeth that have DDE are more likely to be sensitive and consequently providing effective analgesia is often more difficult than for unaffected teeth.

Behavior Management

Clinicians should evaluate the understanding and coping skills of the child with DDE when the teeth require intervention. One of the commonly encountered problems is that children with DDE present with higher levels of anxiety. This is especially true in cases where the defect is associated with sensitivity or where previous treatment has been attempted without appropriate pain control or behavior management. If such defects are suspected, especially when associated with sensitivity, it is important not to air-dry these teeth during examination but to dry them gently with a cotton pellet. Managing young children requires empathy and some knowledge of behavior management techniques for children. Many pediatric dentistry textbooks cover useful techniques for helping children cope with restorative care. In the center of all the techniques is "tell, show, and do" which will allow most children to be able to cooperate for restorative care when it is presented in age-appropriate language and demonstration. This of course takes a little extra time but is time well spent in preparing a child for more complex care as they grow older.

Local Analgesia

For children who have been sensitized to previous invasive dental treatment, in particular local analgesia, the use of computer-controlled anesthesia (such as the Wand and the Wand STA – controlled dental anesthesia, Dental Practice Systems, Welwyn, Herts,

UK) can be an excellent way to administer local analgesia. The Wand provides several advantages over conventional syringes including the fact that it does not look like a conventional syringe; the fine bevel of the needle and the slow speed with which the local analgesic solution can be administered make it a simple way to deliver painless local analgesia. The use of 4 % articaine should be considered in managing older children especially where there is a history of failed local analgesia. For children over 4 years-of-age who are extremely wary of local analgesia, infiltration with 4 % articaine in the lower arch as opposed to an inferior dental block may provide adequate analgesia for restorations to be placed [9]. It is also important to make use of topical anesthesia. The preemptive use of systemic analgesics (in accordance with local guidelines) can also be an effective way of helping children cope with care successfully [10].

Sedation

In extremely apprehensive children who are otherwise cooperative, the use of inhalation sedation should be considered. This form of sedation has the particular benefit of having an analgesic effect which lessens the child's response to painful stimuli. Hence for children whose apprehension is due to sensitive teeth that have been previously treated without effective local analgesia, inhalation sedation with nitrous oxide and oxygen provides a safe, effective, and noninvasive method for managing the child's anxiety [11]. Other forms of sedation can be utilized according to local guidelines and clinicians' usual practice.

General Anesthesia

Clinicians treating children with severe enamel defects should consider the early use of general anesthesia to allow effective successful stabilization of the primary teeth. Previous studies of treatment under general anesthesia have shown good outcomes with decrease in the numbers of repeat restorations [12]. Children with severe enamel defects often present before they are old enough to cope with restorative dentistry; therefore, the use of general anesthesia is effective and valid for this group.

Restorative Management of DDE in the Primary Dentition

The decision to provide restorative management of enamel defects in primary teeth depends on several factors:

1. Type of enamel defect. AI is a generalized condition affecting the entire crown in addition to often being more severe than other developmental defects. The type of AI will also affect the type of restoration provided. Where there is missing enamel or enamel loss after eruption, full-coverage restorations should be considered early in the planning.

2. Extent and severity of the defects. In some cases of chronological hypoplasia, children may have few if any symptoms or significant tooth surface loss, which will suggest that less radical restorative options can be considered.
3. Associated symptoms. In cases of severe sensitivity, full coverage should be considered.
4. Esthetics with possible psychological effects on the child. The psychological impact of these conditions in children should never be underestimated (see Chap. 7). Esthetic management should be offered as soon as the child and the parents wish to have this carried out.
5. Patient cooperation and the method of treatment. In children who cannot cope with treatment under local analgesia, alternative strategies such as sedation or general anesthesia should be considered [7].

Interim Restorations

In some cases it may be appropriate to place interim therapeutic restorations to immediately alleviate pain and sensitivity while awaiting more definitive restorative treatment. The provision of these interim restorations also allows the clinician to establish rapport with the child and assist in behavior management. Materials such as resin-modified glass ionomer can be useful as these materials incorporate appropriate bonding for both enamel and any exposed dentin (Fig. 10.4) [13]. Some of the materials also incorporate a color that allows good visualization of the extent of the restoration on the tooth surface, e.g., Fuji VII/Triage (GC Corporation). The release of fluoride from these materials, although not proven to be a major factor, may also help to reduce sensitivity by encouraging further mineralization of the surrounding enamel. Compomer materials (polyacid-modified composite) might also be considered and can be placed using self-etching primers. These materials have the advantage of being more wear resistant than glass ionomer cement-based materials and have dual-bonding technology, which may seal both enamel and dentin effectively especially when further sealed with adhesive resin or fissure sealant following placement [13].

Longer-Term Restorations of Molar Teeth

Composite Resin Restorations

Composite resin should be considered in cases where:

- The defect is demarcated to a defined area, no more than two surfaces
- Cusp tips are not involved
- There is no significant sensitivity
- Margins of the defect are supragingival

Fig. 10.4 (**a**, **b**) Example of the use of a glass ionomer cement used for interim protection on hypoplastic second primary molars in a 3-year-old (Courtesy of Nicky Kilpatrick)

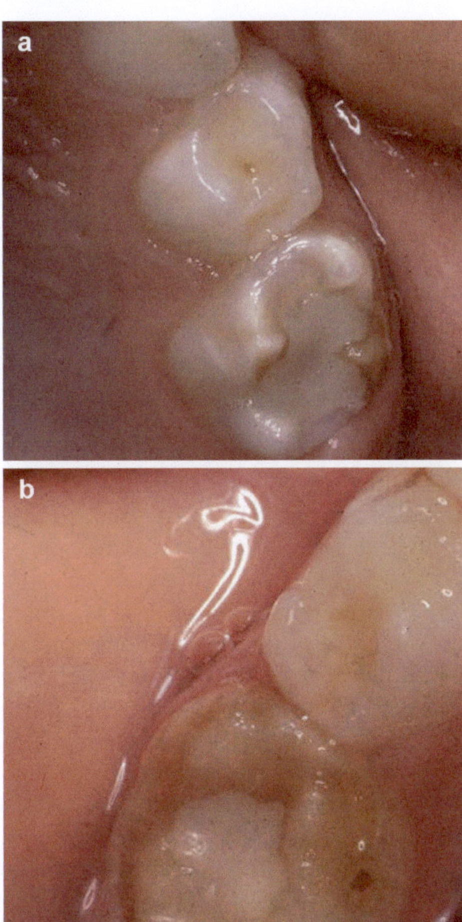

There is evidence to suggest that hypomineralized enamel does not always show a typical etch pattern compared with normal enamel. This can potentially reduce the strength and integrity bond of enamel to composite resin [14, 15]. This is less of an issue with mild cases where normal enamel is present around isolated lesions. Pretreatment with 5 % sodium hypochlorite has been advocated to improve bond strength to hypocalcified enamel [16, 17]. The removal of affected enamel and bonding to dentin, which may be sclerotic, has also been suggested. However research outcomes are still not clear on the most reliable approach to bonding to sclerotic dentine in primary teeth. Recent research would suggest that reduced etching times may result in more reliable bonding particularly when using a total-etch system [18]. Clinicians may need to try different approaches to achieve good results and reviewing research on the particular bonding system being used when planning treatment can be very helpful.

Preformed Crowns

Full coverage with either stainless steel or other esthetic preformed crowns should be considered in cases where:

- The defect involves multiple surfaces.
- There is significant sensitivity.
- Margins of defects are subgingival.
- There is involvement of the cusp tips in posterior teeth.
- Enamel is prone to "chipping," especially in some cases of AI.
- Treatment has to be carried out under general anesthesia and the child is unlikely to manage restorative care in the immediate future.

While preformed metal crowns (stainless steel crowns) are a well-recognized option for the treatment of carious primary molars, they also have an important role in the management of DDE-affected primary molars [19] (Figs. 10.3, 10.5, 10.6, and 10.7). Figures 10.3 and 10.5 illustrate good occlusal support provided by stainless steel crowns. The placement of stainless steel crowns requires minimal tooth preparation. They are less bulky than the white preformed crowns that may suffer wear and chipping of the veneer (Fig. 10.8). More recently for very young children, a technique, known as the "Hall Technique," has been described in which stainless steel crowns are placed with no preparation (Fig. 10.7) [20]. While this technique is promoted for children presenting with dental caries, anecdotal reports suggest that using this technique to place stainless steel crowns over hypomineralized or hypoplastic primary second molars soon after they erupt is a successful way of managing these teeth. Furthermore adopting this technique means that young children can be treated, without resorting to general anesthesia, early in the dental chair without local analgesia. Long-term studies of the use of stainless steel crowns for carious teeth would suggest that crowns placed over teeth with DDE have advantages over other restorative materials [21]:

1. Perform better where more than two surfaces are affected.
2. Less tooth removal is required.
3. Failure rate is much less than other restorative materials.
4. Moisture control is less critical than when restoring with other materials.
5. Placement is less time consuming than resin restorations.
6. Are more cost effective as shown by the outcomes over time.

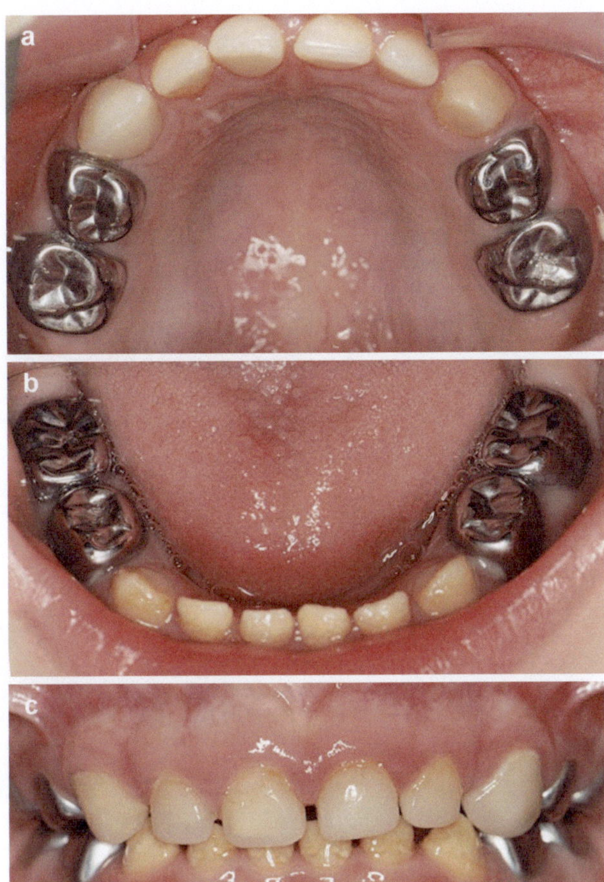

Fig. 10.5 (**a–c**) Intraoral images of same child in Fig. 10.1 with hypoplastic AI, 2 years post-comprehensive restorative care under general anesthetic. Note the significant improvement in gingival health brought about by reduction in sensitivity (Courtesy of Nicky Kilpatrick)

Longer-Term Restorations of Anterior Teeth

Composite restorations are appropriate when restoring anterior teeth with demarcated defects affecting a maximum of two surfaces. Where lesions are diffuse, are large, involve multiple surfaces, or are associated with sensitivity, the use of strip crowns or preformed crowns is advocated [22, 23]. The technique for placing strip crowns involves the removal of approximately 1–2 mm of enamel from all the surfaces of the crown. The enamel is etched and prepared for bonding according to the manufacturer's instructions and the crown is filled with composite, placed on the tooth, with excess removed from the margins and the composite cured. Once the strip crown has

Fig. 10.6 (**a**) Preoperative photograph of child with hypomaturation-hypoplasia AI. (**b**) Postoperative photograph showing restoration of the hypoplastic second primary molars using stainless steel crowns. The anterior teeth were mildly affected, asymptomatic, and esthetically acceptable, therefore were managed with preventive care

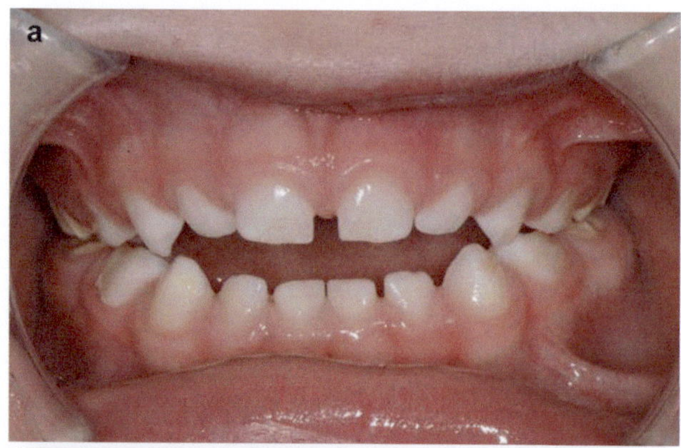

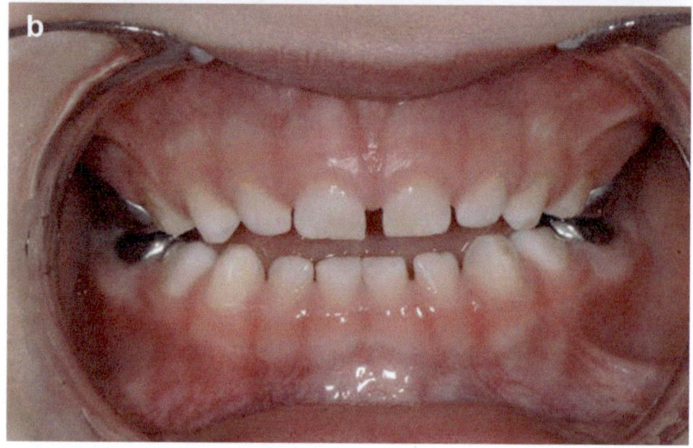

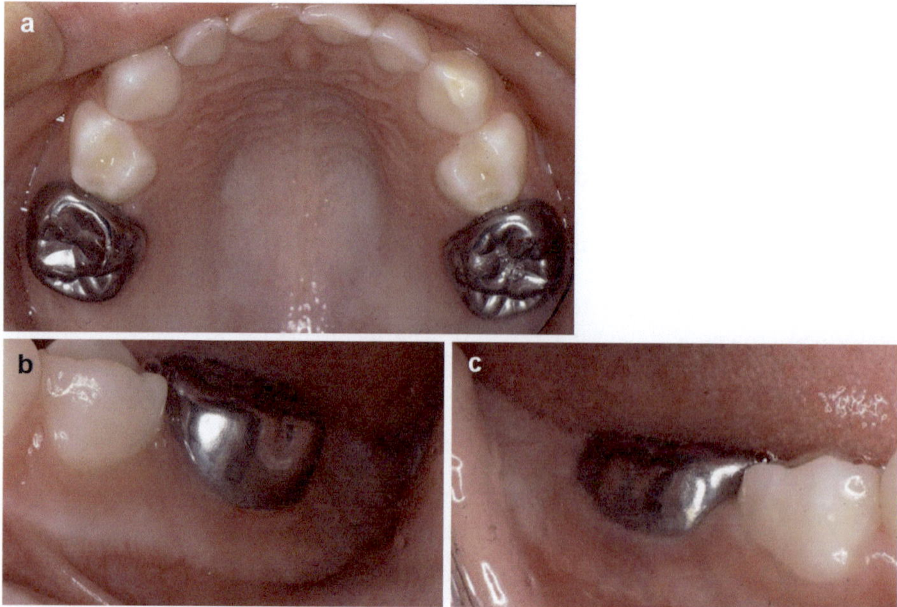

Fig. 10.7 (**a–c**) Same child as in Fig. 10.4 post-placement of stainless steel crowns on second primary molars using the Hall technique (Courtesy of Nicky Kilpatrick)

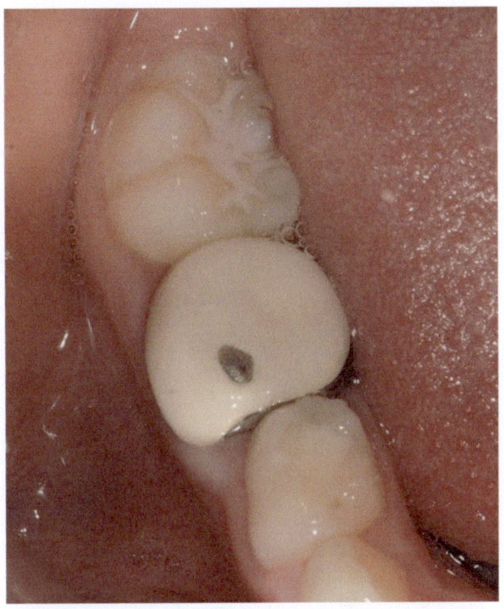

Fig. 10.8 Occlusal view showing restoration of the lower right second primary molar with NuSmile Signature white crown in which the veneer has chipped but the crown remains intact

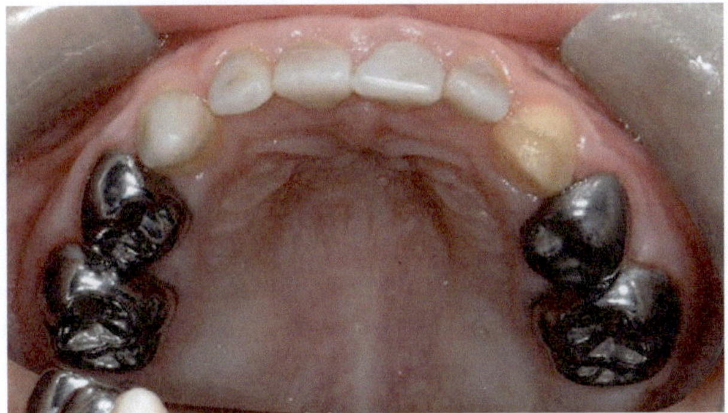

Fig. 10.9 Occlusal view of anterior strip crowns and stainless steel crowns placed in a child with AI (Courtesy of Nicky Kilpatrick)

been removed, the restoration is finished in the usual manner (Figs. 10.5c and 10.9). More recently, the use of preformed white veneered crowns such as NuSmile Signature and pre-veneered Kinder Krowns® or zirconia crowns such as NuSmile zirconia and Zirconia Anterior Kinder Krowns® is advocated by some clinicians. These crowns provide very good esthetic results (Fig. 10.10). However they do require more extensive crown preparation and care must be taken to protect the pulp. The preformed crowns do have a higher cost and chipping can occur in the veneered stainless steel crowns (Fig. 10.8). Further studies are needed to assess the longevity of these restorations with particular attention being paid to their cost-effectiveness.

Extraction of Primary Teeth with DDE

In some cases extractions of severely affected teeth may be required. This should be done with evaluation of the space requirements in the developing dentition. In children where multiple teeth are affected and extractions are required, an

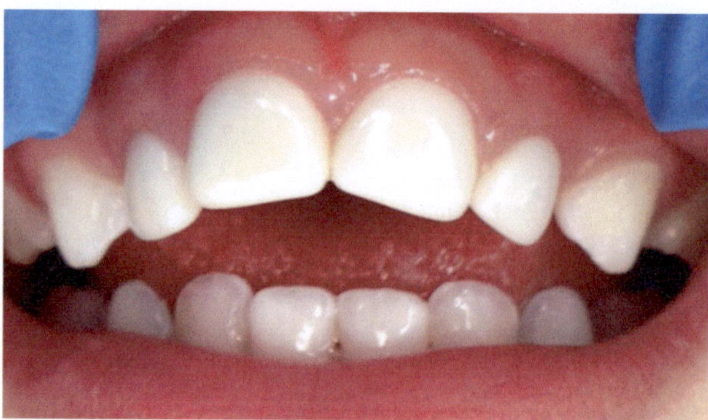

Fig. 10.10 Anterior primary incisors with zirconia crowns in a 2-year-old child (Courtesy of Bernadette Drummond)

interdisciplinary approach involving an orthodontist should be considered to optimize the development of the permanent dentition occlusion. Wherever possible, preventive and restorative approaches should be the preferred option as this always gives the child and their family a positive dental health message, where preservation of teeth is considered important. For further discussion regarding the interdisciplinary treatment planning needed for these children, see Chap. 8.

Summary

Children who suffer from DDE in their primary dentition deserve the highest quality restorative and preventive treatment. These children can be young, extremely apprehensive, and often caries-free, which means that management of affected teeth may be their first experience of invasive dentistry. Treatment should be provided with the use of appropriate behavior management techniques and analgesia to help children develop skills to cope with the restorative care both immediately and into their future.

References

1. Seow W, Brown J, Tudehope D, O'Callaghan M. Developmental defects in the primary dentition of low birth-weight infants: adverse effects of laryngoscopy and prolonged endotracheal intubation. Pediatr Dent. 1984;6:28–31.
2. Pindborg J. Aetiology of developmental enamel defects not related to fluorosis. Int Dent J. 1982;32:123–4.
3. Poulsen S, Gjørup H, Haubek D, Haukali G, Hintze H, Løvschall H, et al. Amelogenesis imperfecta – a systematic literature review of associated dental and oro-facial abnormalities and their impact on patients. Acta Odontol Scand. 2008;66(4):193–9.
4. Welbury R, Gillgrass T. Craniofacial growth and development. In: Welbury R, Duggal M, Hosey M, editors. Paediatric dentistry. 4th ed. Oxford: Oxford University Press; 2012. p. 12–3. Chapter 1.
5. Gadhia K, McDonald S, Arkutu N, Malik K. Amelogenesis imperfecta: an introduction. Br Dent J. 2012;212:377–9.

6. McDonald S, Arkutu N, Malik K, Gadhia K, McKaig S. Managing the paediatric patient with amelogenesis imperfecta. Br Dent J. 2012;212(9):425–8.

7. Jälevik B, Klingberg G. Dental treatment, dental fear and behaviour management problems in children with severe enamel hypomineralization of their first permanent molars. Int J Paediatr Dent. 2002;12:24–32.

8. Department of Health and British Association for the study of Community Dentistry. Delivering better oral health. An evidence-based toolkit for prevention. London; 2009.

9. Leith R, Lynch K, O'Connell A. Articaine use in children: a review. Eur Arch Paediatr Dent. 2012;13(6):293–6.

10. Baygin O, Tuzuner T, Isik B, Kusgoz A, Tanriver M. Comparison of pre-emptive ibuprofen, paracetamol, and placebo administration in reducing post-operative pain in primary tooth extraction. Int J Paediatr Dent. 2011;21(4):306–13.

11. Paterson SA, Tahmassebi JF. Paediatric dentistry in the new millennium: 3. Use of inhalation sedation in paediatric dentistry. Dent Update. 2003;30:350–8.

12. Drummond B, Davidson L, Williams S, Moffat S, Ayers K. Outcomes two, three and four years after comprehensive care under general anaesthesia. N Z Dent J. 2004;100(2):32–7.

13. Gjorgievska E, Nicholson J, Iljovska S, Slipper I. Marginal adaptation and performance of bioactive dental restorative materials in deciduous and young permanent teeth. J Appl Oral Sci. 2008;16(1):1–6.

14. Mahoney E, Ismail FS, et al. Mechanical properties across hypomineralized/hypoplastic enamel of first permanent molar teeth. Eur J Oral Sci. 2004;112(6):497–502.

15. William V, Burrow M, Palamara J, Messer L. Microshear bond strength of resin composite to teeth affected by molar hypomineralization using 2 adhesive systems. Pediatr Dent. 2006;28:233–41.

16. Şaroğlu IAŞ, Öztaş D. Effect of deproteinization on composite bond strength in hypocalcified amelogenesis imperfecta. Oral Dis. 2006;12(3):305–8.

17. Venezie R, Vadiakas G, Christensen J, Wright J. Enamel pretreatment with sodium hypochlorite to enhance bonding in hypocalcified amelogenesis imperfecta: case report and SEM analysis. Pediatr Dent. 1994;16(6):433–6.

18. Osorio R, Aguilera F, Otero P, Romero M, Osorio E, Garcia-Godoy F, et al. Primary dentin etching time, bond strength and ultra-structure characterization of dentin surfaces. J Dent. 2010;38(3):222–31.

19. Kindelan S, Day P, Nichol R, Willmott N, Fayle S. UK national clinical guidelines in paediatric dentistry: stainless steel preformed crowns for primary molars. Int J Paediatr Dent. 2008;18 Suppl 1:20–8.

20. Innes N, Evans D, Hall N. The Hall technique for managing carious primary molars. Dent Update. 2009;36(8):472–4. 7–8.

21. Attari NRJ. Restoration of primary teeth with crowns: a systematic review of the literature. Eur Arch Paediatr Dent. 2006;7(2):58–62.

22. Webber D, Epstein N, Wong J, Tsamtsouris A. A method of restoring primary anterior teeth with the aid of a celluloid crown form and composite resins. Pediatr Dent. 1979;1(4):244–6.

23. Kupietzky A, Waggoner W, Galea J. Long-term photographic and radiographic assessment of bonded resin composite strip crowns for primary incisors: results after 3 years. Pediatr Dent. 2005;27:221–5.

Restorative Management of Permanent Teeth Enamel Defects in Children and Adolescents

11

Suzanne M. Hanlin, Lucy A.L. Burbridge, and Bernadette K. Drummond

Abstract

The clinical challenges associated with the restorative management of developmental defects of enamel (DDE) have been well documented and include managing sensitivity and caries risk, loss of occlusal determinants, and the negative impact on individual self-worth and social interaction. This chapter outlines management options for DDE associated with molar incisor hypomineralization (MIH), amelogenesis imperfecta (AI), fluorosis, and intrinsic discoloration in permanent teeth. Many materials and techniques may be used to manage DDE. The complexity of intervention is dictated by the severity and nature of the disturbances including color (brown/cream/yellow/white opacities – hypomineralization), structure (hypoplasia – pits, grooves), pre-eruptive resorption, post-eruptive breakdown, the patient's individual circumstances, and the age and stage of development.

S.M. Hanlin, BDS, MDS, GradDipHealInf
Department of Oral Rehabilitation, Faculty of Dentistry, University of Otago, PO Box 647, 9054 Dunedin, New Zealand
e-mail: suzanne.hanlin@otago.ac.nz

L.A.L. Burbridge, BDS DipConSed, MClinDent
Paediatric Dental Department, Newcastle Dental Hospital, Newcastle Upon Tyne NE2 4AZ, UK
e-mail: lucy.burbridge@nuth.nhs.uk

B.K. Drummond, BDS, MS, PhD (✉)
Department of Oral Sciences, Faculty of Dentistry, University of Otago, 310 Great King Street, PO Box 647, Dunedin 9054, New Zealand
e-mail: bernadette.drummond@otago.ac.nz

© Springer-Verlag Berlin Heidelberg 2015

139

B.K. Drummond, N. Kilpatrick (eds.), *Planning and Care for Children and Adolescents with Dental Enamel Defects: Etiology, Research and Contemporary Management*, DOI 10.1007/978-3-662-44800-7_11

Introduction

The aim of treatment for a child or adolescent with developmental defects of enamel (DDE) is to provide comfort, natural form, and function and prevent additional problems. Setting achievable goals is key to ensuring a successful outcome because the impact on perception of attractiveness and well-being can sometimes skew and heighten the expectations of children and families unrealistically [1]. Management and maintenance costs can be considerable and impact directly and indirectly on all members of a family. Extensive defects may be associated with other anomalies and the development of an interdisciplinary plan in early childhood is important to protect compromised tooth structure and establish occlusal stability [2]. Definitive management may not occur until late adolescence or early adulthood, and consideration must be given to the ability of children to manage treatment and avoid burnout. Clinicians must be responsive to the changing esthetic and functional needs of the developing child and adolescent.

Restorative modalities can include tooth bleaching and microabrasion therapy, enamel infiltration with composite resin [3], direct and indirect veneering materials and/or indirect (laboratory-fabricated or computer-aided design, CAD-milled) polymethyl methacrylate (PMMA), and composite or ceramic restorations. Full-coverage restorations may be required for more severely affected teeth where masking of the underlying tooth color is required, or there is severe sensitivity or a need to improve the shape of the tooth. Preformed stainless steel crowns (SSC) can be placed on affected permanent (as well as primary) molar teeth in childhood to maintain occlusal support and arch length [4]. The use of composite, acrylic, or polycarbonate shell crowns has also been reported [5, 6]. In late adolescence or early adulthood, these interim solutions may be replaced with laboratory-fabricated composite resin, ceramic, porcelain fused to metal (PFM), cast, or CAD-milled ceramic or alloy crowns.

Choosing Materials and Techniques for Bonding in Compromised Enamel

Because of the wide variation in the clinical presentation of enamel defects, recognition of the etiology and subsequent management can be difficult. However, differential diagnosis of the defect will assist in determining which treatment techniques and materials may perform best. It has been suggested that by understanding the origin of the enamel defect, clinicians are able to more appropriately target the treatment to the patient's needs, preserve residual tooth structure, and avoid overly invasive procedures [7]. Conventional enamel etching and bonding techniques following manufacturer's guidelines are usually successful for enamel that is reduced in quantity but still well mineralized (i.e., thin or hypoplastic). If dentine is relatively unaffected, dentine bonding systems, glass ionomer, polyacid-modified composite resins (PMCR), or resin-modified glass ionomer cements

(RMGIC) offer predictable bond strengths to dentine and improve restoration prognosis. Hypomineralized enamel and/or a defective dentinoenamel junction (DEJ) affects the restoration bond strength, and the enamel may shear off or detach. Hypocalcified enamel often results in increased wear rates and chipping. Hypomineralized enamel (containing more protein) exhibits significantly lower micro-shear bond strengths with predominantly cohesive fractures of restorations and enamel loss due to shallow etching patterns, a porous adhesive interface, and cracks in the enamel [8].

Approaches that have been investigated to improve bonding to defective enamel include modification of the acid used for etching (organic rather than inorganic), use of self-etching primers, glass ionomer cement sandwiches with composite, resin-modified glass ionomer cements (RMGIC), and pretreatment of enamel with 5 % sodium hypochlorite [9–15]. However to date, none of these approaches provide a predictable way of achieving adhesion to hypomineralized enamel. This remains a challenge for long-term restoration success and is probably the single most important factor that forces progression to full-coverage restorations in late adolescence or early adulthood.

Management of Enamel Defects in Anterior Teeth

Treatment of anterior teeth with enamel defects is usually initiated by patients because of dissatisfaction with their appearance. Improvement is important for psychosocial well-being particularly during the mixed and early permanent dentitions [16, 17] (See Chap. 7). During childhood, the least invasive approach necessary to meet the esthetic demands of each individual should be adopted. For every technique, pretreatment radiographs and tooth shades should be recorded at baseline against which changes can be assessed over the long term.

Microabrasion

Acid pumice microabrasion is a controlled method of removing surface enamel to reduce discolorations particularly when this is limited to superficial layers and to allow further mineralization. Microabrasion is achieved by a combination of abrasion and erosion ("abrosion") [18]. Approximately 100 μm of enamel is removed in one or two appointments. Any additional enamel removal has the potential to damage the pulp or can result in exposure of underlying dentine [19].

Indications
- Diffuse (superficial) and small demarcated enamel opacities
- Hypomineralized enamel defects
- Post-orthodontic treatment decalcification
- Initial treatment for demarcated enamel opacities

Contraindications
- Deep hypoplastic enamel defects
- Intrinsic discolorations, e.g., tetracycline (dentinal) discoloration
- Discoloration associated with nonvital teeth

Technique
- Clean teeth with pumice and water to remove superficial staining and plaque and expose a clean enamel surface, wash, and dry.
- Isolate the teeth with dental dam. Mix 18 % hydrochloric acid (HCl) with pumice into a slurry or use acid from a proprietary kit. Apply a small amount to the labial surfaces using a rubber cup rotating slowly (5–10 s). Wash carefully into an aspirator tip. Repeat until the stain has reduced, up to a maximum of 60-s acid exposure. Remove the dam and apply color-free neutral fluoride.
- The patient should apply either fluoride gel- or a calcium-based material (CCP–ACP, calcium triphosphate) several times a day until follow-up to enhance remineralization.
- Review 2–4 weeks later, repeat once more if clinically indicated, and if not, consider an alternative treatment modality. Repeat sensibility tests and update photographs.

Outcome

It is important to give detailed preoperative explanation to establish realistic expectations. Delay final review for at least 1 month as the appearance of the teeth will continue to improve over this time [20]. The best outcomes are achieved in cases of brown mottling that are more easily masked than more opaque white lesions and even white mottling becomes less perceptible (Fig. 11.1a, b). Improvement has been attributed to the relatively prismless layer of compacted surface enamel produced by the "abrosion" technique which alters the optical properties of the tooth surface [18]. No associations between microabrasion and pulpal damage, increased caries susceptibility, or prolonged thermal sensitivity have been reported. The technique is straightforward and not time-consuming to perform for the operator or patient. Microabrasion may assist with masking of a lesion in preparation for later composite restorations or veneers. This technique can be used in conjunction with bleaching agents with good outcomes [21] and can reduce the impact of the yellow hue or lighten other staining further [22, 23].

Bleaching

A bleaching agent (e.g., 10 % carbamide peroxide) can be applied to the surfaces of teeth with the aim being to lighten color. The exact mechanism of bleaching is unknown, but the release of hydrogen peroxide anions, reactive oxygen molecules, and free radicals is thought to be involved in lightening the stained mineral and

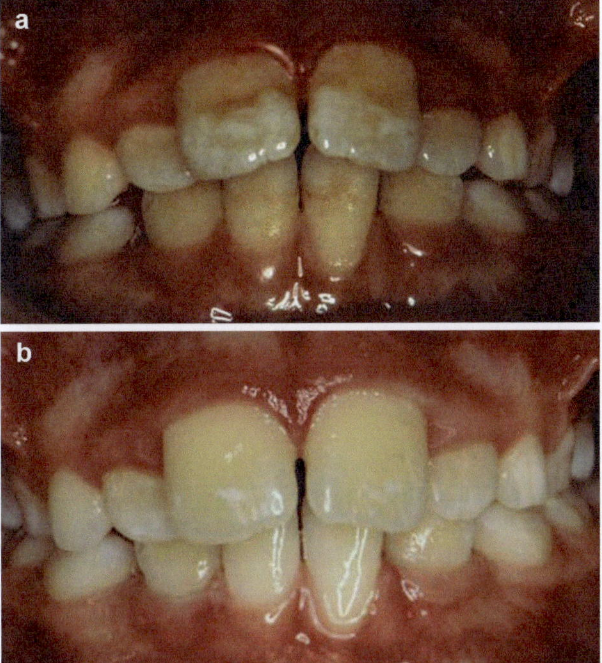

Fig. 11.1 (**a, b**) Change in enamel on permanent upper incisors following two microabrasion treatments with ongoing use of CPP-ACP with fluoride

protein in the enamel. Discoloration can reoccur because of a combination of chemical reduction of the previously formed oxidation products, marginal leakage of restorations allowing ingress of bacterial and chemical by-products, salivary or tissue fluid contamination, or food color contamination via the permeable tooth structure.

Indications
- Hypomineralized enamel defects
- Mild tetracycline staining
- Mild fluorosis

Contraindications
- Hypoplastic enamel defects

Techniques
- Vital bleaching can occur chairside/in the office or at home using custom-designed bleaching trays (vacuum formed).
- The in-office technique involves application of carbamide peroxide to the surfaces of the teeth with activation of the process by a heat source. This consumes chair time, adding to the expense. It is useful for treatment of mild enamel defects where strict isolation of a single tooth is required.

- The home bleaching technique utilizes a custom bleaching tray constructed for the maxillary and/or the mandibular teeth. The patient applies the carbamide peroxide (gel) to the teeth via the tray on a daily basis until the desired color change is achieved. There are many proprietary products available, and the principal differences lie in the concentration of carbamide peroxide employed and the amount of hydrogen peroxide released. Current recommendations indicate that a 10 % solution is both safe and successful in modifying tooth color.
- The concurrent use of a calcium-based product such as that with casein phospho-peptide–amorphous calcium phosphate will control any tooth sensitivity.
- Review 2–6 weeks later. An 80 % color change should have occurred.
- Take postoperative photographs including the pre- and posttreatment shade tab for long-term records.

Outcome

Minor ulceration or irritation may occur during the initial treatment which may relate to tray overextension. There may be transient pulpal sensitivity because carbamide peroxide gel (10 %) breaks down in the mouth into 3 % hydrogen peroxide and 7 % urea. Both have low molecular weights that allow them to diffuse through enamel and dentine and cause pulp irritation [24]. If sensitivity occurs, exposure time can be decreased, or it may be necessary to discontinue treatment. To date, there is no evidence that bleaching solutions with a low pH (below the critical pH of 5.2–5.8) causes enamel demineralization [25], possibly because urea, followed by ammonia and carbon dioxide, is released on degradation of the carbamide peroxide elevating the pH. Bond strength of composite resin to bleached enamel decreases initially and has been attributed to the residual oxygen in the bleached tooth surface inhibiting polymerization of the composite resin, but this returns to normal within 7 days [26]. Vital-bleaching systems do not modify the color of restorative materials and any perceived effect is probably due to superficial cleansing. Regular retreatment may be necessary to maintain effective lightening [27]. When considering the use of bleaching products, the clinicians should be mindful of local regulations and seek advice with respect to contemporary legislation.

Direct Restoration with Composite Resin

Composite resin bonded to etched enamel and/or pretreated dentine can be used to restore tooth defects or improve esthetics by replacing or masking areas of discolored or defective enamel.

Indications
- Demarcated enamel opacities
- Hypoplastic enamel defects

Contraindications
- Diffuse enamel opacities

Technique
- Apply dental dam and contoured matrix strips if required.
- Selective removal of demarcated lesion with a round diamond bur may be required to optimize esthetics and bonding; however, bonding can also be improved by selective use of GIC, or polyacid-modified composite.
- The enamel margins can be chamfered with a diamond fissure bur to increase the surface area for retention and blend the composite margin with the enamel.
- Etch the area, wash and dry, and apply the primer, bonding agent, and the chosen shade of composite. A brush lubricated with bonding agent can be used to smooth and shape before light curing.
- Remove the matrix strip/dam, polish with graded polishing discs and diamond finishing burs, and characterize the surface if required.
- Take postoperative photographs for records. .

Outcomes

Restoration of localized hypomineralized or hypoplastic defects using composite resin is not usually associated with sensitivity and may not need local anesthesia unless there is caries with extension into dentine. These very conservative resin-bonded restorations are particularly suited to newly erupted incisors (Fig. 11.2a, b).

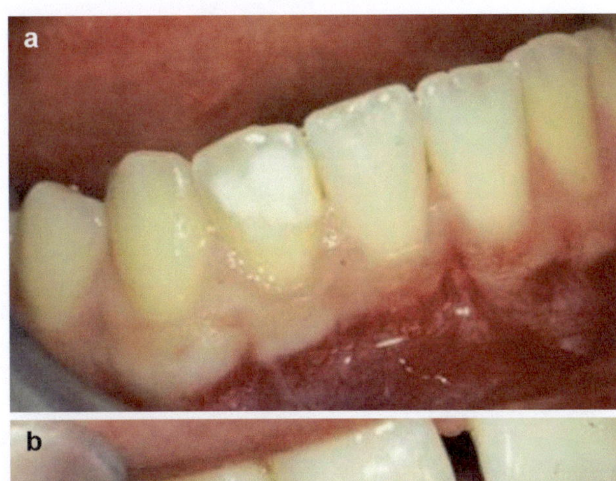

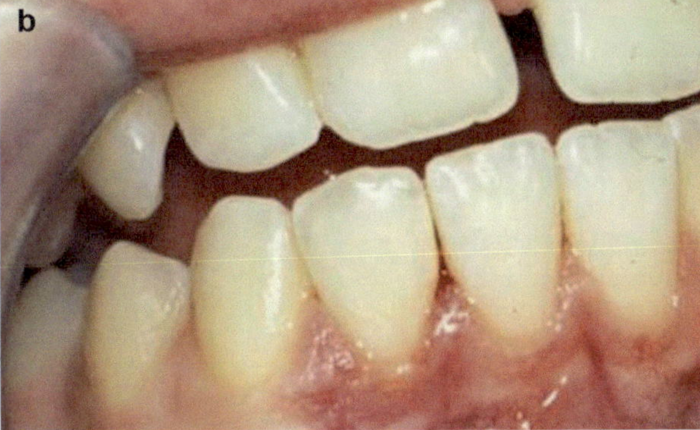

Fig. 11.2 (**a**, **b**) Lesion on the lower right lateral incisor masked with composite resin

However, when it is not possible or desirable to remove the entire opacity, problems with marginal staining, color matching, and suboptimal esthetics can arise.

Composite Resin Veneers

Composite resin can be used as a veneer to cover the entire labial aspect of the tooth and improve color and contour. These veneers can also protect against further breakdown of severely hypoplastic enamel as shown in Fig. 11.3a, b. Composite veneers may be directly placed at the chairside or indirectly fabricated in the laboratory. Composite veneering is conservative, cost-effective, and repairable in the mouth and may offer a satisfactory long-term alternative to full-coverage restoration in mild enamel defects even in adults. They are useful in the young dentition, in immature teeth with large pulp horns, large pulp chambers, immature gingival contour, and short crown height on teeth that are still erupting.

Before proceeding with any veneering technique, it is necessary to decide whether to reduce the thickness of labial enamel. Increased labio-palatal bulk without tooth preparation makes it harder to maintain good oral hygiene. However, increase in the labial contour may enhance appearance of in-standing or rotated

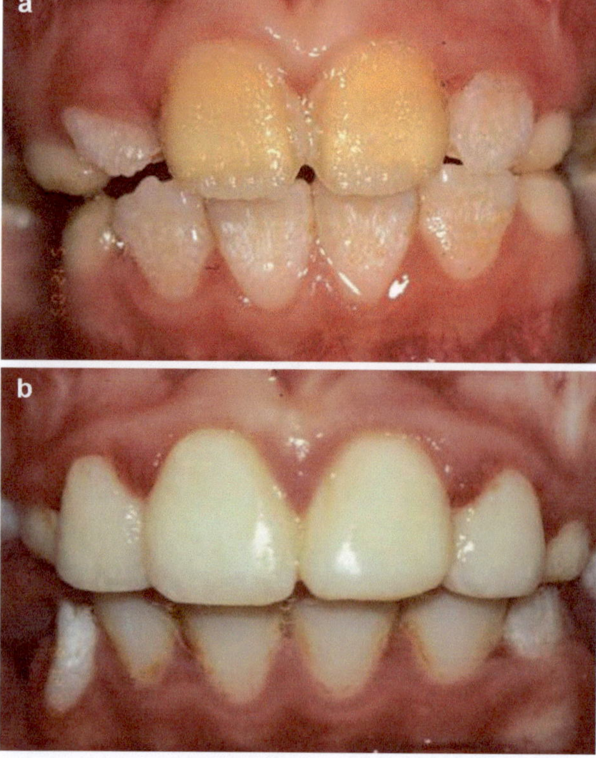

Fig. 11.3 (**a, b**) Resin veneers for upper incisors in the early mixed dentition period

teeth. Bond strengths to enamel are increased when 200–300 μm of the surface enamel is removed, and the restoration will maintain the tooth contour. Some reduction and/or use of an opaquing agent may be required to mask intense stain in a discolored tooth. Hybrid composite resins finished to a higher surface luster can replace relatively large amounts of missing tooth tissue or may be used in thin sections. Layering of dentine and enamel shades can be used to simulate natural color gradations and hues.

Indications
- Large demarcated enamel opacities
- Widespread hypoplastic enamel defects

Contraindications
- Very darkly discolored teeth
- Minimal enamel defects
- Insufficient tooth tissue available for bonding
- Oral habits, e.g., woodwind musicians where embrasure may be critical
- Heavy occlusal load/parafunction

Technique: Direct Composite Veneers
- Use a tapered diamond or sharp tungsten carbide bur to reduce labial enamel by 0.3–0.5 mm if required. Identify a finish line at the gingival margin and extend mesially and distally just labial to the contact points.
- Clean with a slurry of pumice in water, wash, and dry to remove plaque and debris.
- Isolate the tooth with dam and a contoured matrix strip if needed.
- Etch enamel, wash, and dry. Apply a thin layer of primer and bond with a brush and use an opaquing agent at this stage if discoloration is intense.
- Apply composite resin and shape. Light cure according to manufacturer's instructions at the gingival margin and the mesio-incisal, disto-incisal, and palatal aspects if incisal coverage has been used. Different shades can be combined to achieve matches with adjacent teeth and transition from a relatively darker gingival area to a lighter more translucent incisal region.
- Finish the margins with diamond finishing burs and interproximal strips and the labial surface with graded finishing discs.
- Take postoperative photographs for records.

Outcome

Good esthetics can be maintained for many years with regular reviews and repolishing as needed [28]. Indirect composite veneers can be fabricated from elastomeric impressions of the teeth, direct scanning of the prepared tooth or indirect scanning of a stone working cast. Laboratory-fabricated composite veneers can provide many of the characteristics of a ceramic veneer as described below. Color reproduction and surface wear are improving. However, in a situation with high esthetic demand, porcelain would still be the material of choice for restoration longevity and stability.

Porcelain Veneers

Porcelain has superior esthetic properties to composite resin, improved resistance to abrasion, and is well tolerated by gingival tissues. However, porcelain requires tooth preparation to maximize fit and maintain tooth contour and to allow replication of color. Disadvantages are that it is not repairable in the mouth and the laboratory stages add to cost when compared to directly placed restorations. Best outcomes are obtained after teeth have erupted completely, and therefore these restorations should generally be delayed until late adolescence (ideally after 20 years of age). Further information about preparation and design are covered in prosthodontic textbooks.

Restorative Management of Enamel Defects in Posterior Teeth

Clinicians face challenges when attempting to cover posterior teeth that are partially erupted, have significant sensitivity, suffer post-eruptive breakdown, or are difficult to anesthetize. Recommendations for managing sensitivity are included in Chap. 9. Where it is not appropriate to seal enamel because of the degree of hypomineralization, longer-term solutions are required.

Planning and Trialing the Occlusal Scheme

Patients with isolated teeth affected by enamel defects may have stable intra- (tooth to tooth) and inter-arch (maxilla to mandible) contacts, and acceptable arch alignment and length that provide a functional occlusion. Restorative management can be undertaken while conforming to the existing occlusal scheme. Where there is significant hypoplasia of the occlusal surfaces of molars and premolars, the teeth may not erupt into contact or the occlusal contacts that are formed may be on unstable inclined planes that predispose to tooth movement and tooth chipping. Specific malocclusions are associated with some types of AI including anterior open bite, delayed eruption, and/or missing teeth [29]. In such cases, a reorganized occlusal scheme has to be planned, and the vertical dimension, tooth replacement and repositioning, restorative materials, and techniques all have to be taken in to consideration in order to achieve long-term occlusal stability. Creation of the final occlusal interface requires a restorative solution, but arch alignment, uncovering teeth and preservation of arch length, requires orthodontic and sometimes surgical management to support the restorative plan. Compromises in the ideal plan may often occur with successful management requiring ongoing explanation and discussion with patients and parents.

Where enamel defects are minimal and the teeth have areas of normal enamel, composite resin may be placed on the occlusal surfaces taking care to overlap the bonded margins onto healthy enamel. Preformed stainless steel crowns placed over the tooth with minimal or no preparation provide a very useful intermediate option in the younger child. Before the permanent dentition has erupted, children usually manage well if "bite opening" occurs when crowns are placed. However, care should be taken when there is an existing anterior open bite. In adolescents, other options such as PMMA resin crowns or Zirconia-milled crowns are being trialed where esthetics may be of particular concern.

Stainless Steel Crowns

Stainless steel crowns have proved to be a very successful solution to preserve posterior molars with developmental defects or other defects during childhood and adolescence until an appropriate time to place more permanent restorations.

Indications
- Hypomineralized molars with breakdown or sensitivity
- Hypoplastic molars
- To prevent further tooth wear

Contraindications
- Severely broken down tooth that cannot retain the crown.
- Extraction and orthodontic management is preferred.

Technique with Tooth Preparation
- Provide local anesthesia and systemic analgesia if required for very sensitive teeth.
- Minimally reduce the mesial, distal, and occlusal surfaces with a fine tapered diamond
- Select and fit the appropriate crown. The crown height may need to be reduced, crimped, and polished to place the margin just at the gingival margin of the tooth [30].
- Check the occlusion, remove the crown, fill with a GIC-based cement, and replace other tooth. Have the patient bite on gauze to seat the crown firmly. Remove excess cement. Interproximal cement can be removed with floss with several knots that is pulled through under the contact point.

Technique with No Tooth Preparation
- If possible, place orthodontic separating elastics a few days before treatment.
- Select the appropriate crown and adjust the height if required. Crimp the crown and seat to check the margin.
- Check the occlusion, remove the crown, fill with an appropriate cement, and replace on the tooth. Have the patient bite on gauze to seat the crown firmly. Remove excess cement. Interproximal cement can be removed with floss with several knots pulled through under the contact point.

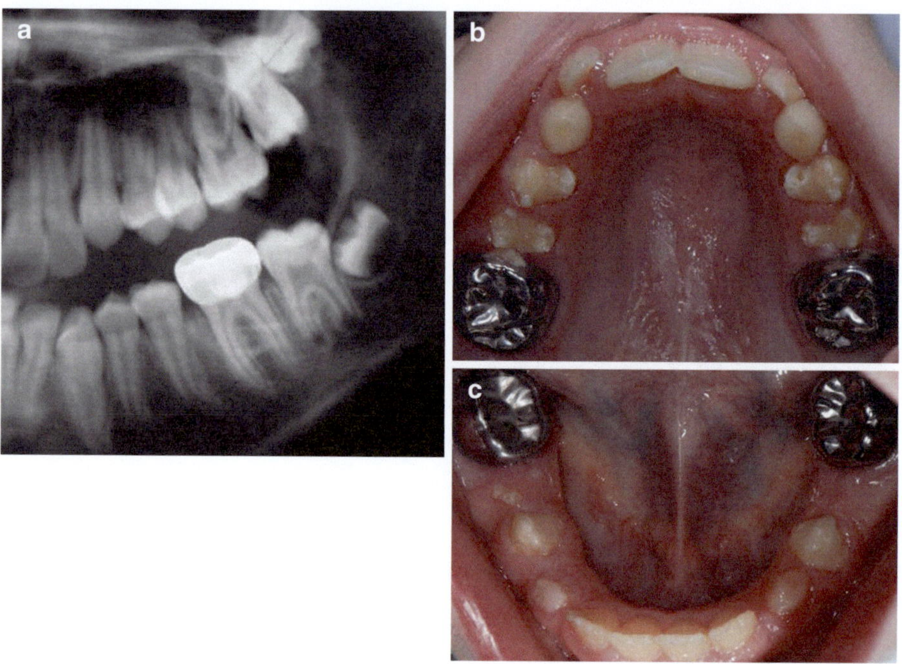

Fig. 11.4 (**a**) Radiographic appearance of appearance of a stainless steel crown on a lower left first molar with DDE. (**b, c**) Stainless steel crowns placed on severely hypoplastic molars in AI. Note the hypoplasia of the rest of the erupting permanent teeth

Outcome

Stainless steel crowns seal the teeth and provide thermal protection allowing the pulps to mature. The enamel is protected from breakdown, the occlusion is maintained, and the teeth can continue to erupt to the mature height, thus providing optimal conditions for more definitive solutions in late adolescence or adulthood [4]. This is illustrated in Fig. 11.4a–c.

Periodontal Management: Gingival Recontouring and Crown Lengthening

Adolescents with gingival enlargement, delayed or failed eruption of teeth or impacted teeth, and missing teeth may require surgical intervention such as gingival recontouring, crown lengthening, or surgical exposure prior to restoration. These can be done using traditional surgical approaches and/or with soft tissue laser surgery which is associated with improved tissue healing and reduced postoperative discomfort [31]. Figure 11.5a–c demonstrates the increase in available enamel that can be created following gingival recontouring in an adolescent with hypoplastic

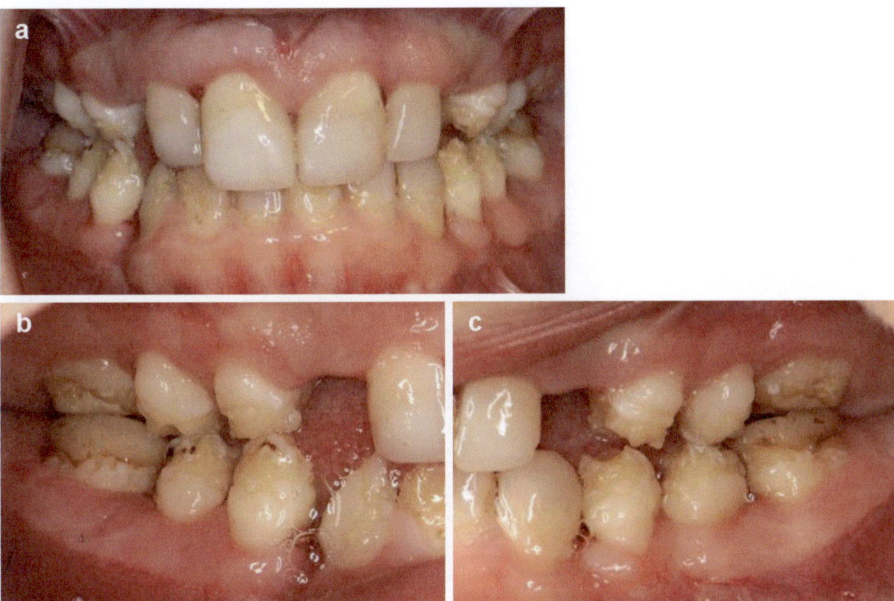

Fig. 11.5 (**a–c**) Post crown lengthening surgery in maxillary and mandibular right and left quadrants showing access to good quality enamel in hypoplastic AI

AI. The extent of the defects and number of teeth will determine if periodontal management can be undertaken with local anesthetic alone or will require sedation or general anesthesia. A team approach involving a pediatric dentist, prosthodontist, periodontist, and orthodontist is important to optimize care. Good explanation of the short- and long-term goals will help children and their parents understand the reasons for surgery and the restorative plan.

Indirect Interim Restorations

Laboratory-fabricated composite resin (CR) crowns, CAD-milled PMMA, or CR provisional crowns constructed from scans of the dentition may be resilient interim restorations during adolescence. Premolar teeth can also be restored with directly or indirectly fabricated composite onlay restorations or with complete coronal recontouring determined by the extent of the enamel defects. Pretreatment diagnostic wax-up of the desired tooth form and contacts is useful in planning for this. Teeth affected by AI may have a rim of less affected enamel at or just below the gingival cuff, and once uncovered this provides a satisfactory finish line, requiring minimal additional tooth preparation for indirectly fabricated restorations (onlays/overlays or crowns). This is illustrated in Fig. 11.6a–c.

Fig. 11.6 (**a–c**) Interim PMMA provisional crowns (splinted on posterior teeth) and directly built composite resin onlays on anterior teeth in preparation for laboratory-fabricated composite resin crowns to provide protection and functional form during orthodontic management. Note missing 13 and 23 failure of eruption

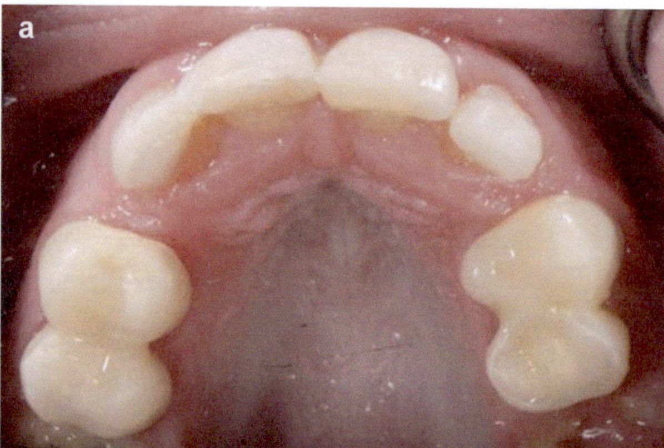

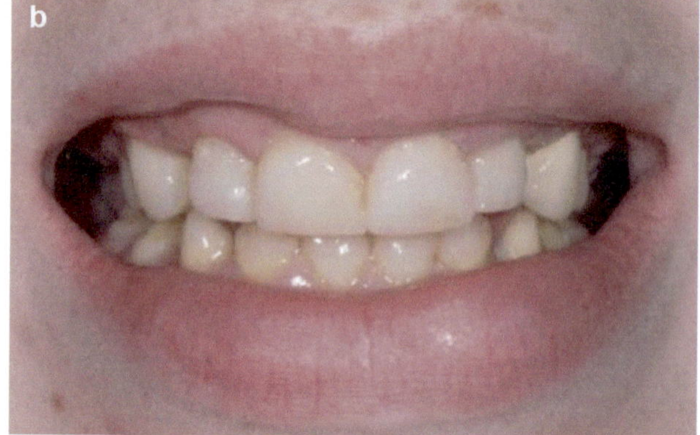

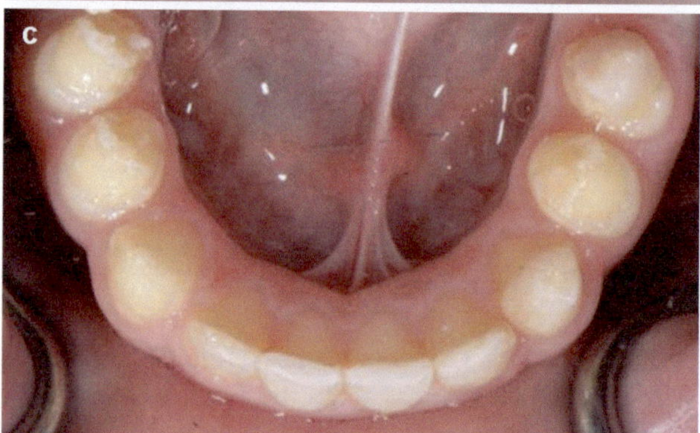

Partial Veneers/Occlusal Overlays and Crowns

Veneers, overlays, or crowns restore missing tooth tissue by surrounding part or all of the remaining natural structure [32]. They restore form, function, esthetics, and longevity and provide protection. They are indicated for teeth with large occlusal

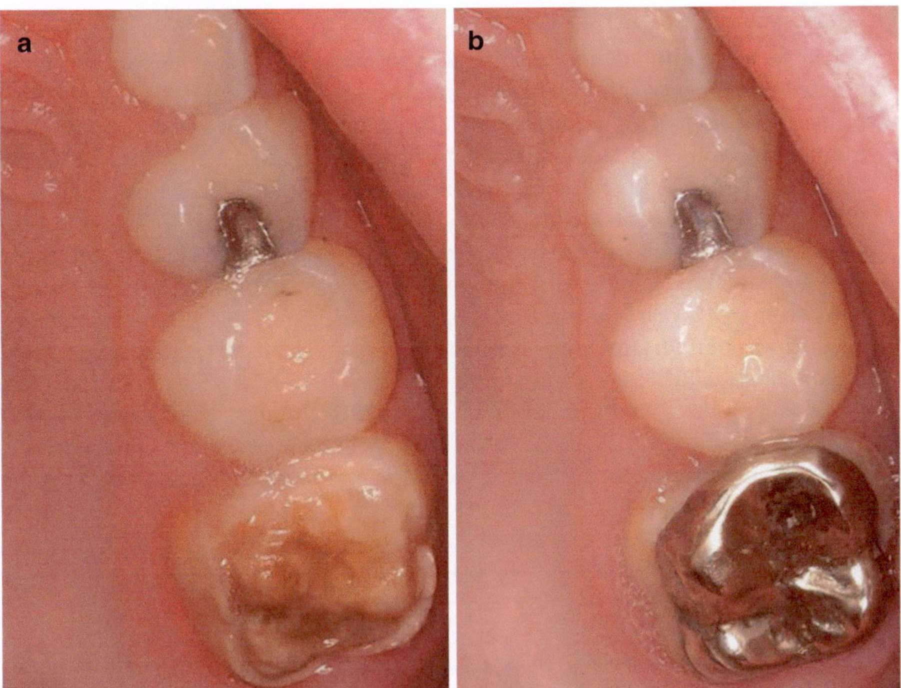

Fig. 11.7 (**a**, **b**) Pre- and post-placement of a preformed gold onlay, cemented on unprepared upper first molar using Panavia Ex

defects and are well described in restorative dentistry textbooks. Limitations include patients who are unable to cooperate for the procedure, financial constraints, compromised pulpal or periodontal prognosis, or lack of adequate supporting dentine. Veneers, overlays, or crowns may be preformed, laboratory fabricated or generated by CAD–CAM technology in either the clinic or laboratory. Many materials are available or in development and include non-precious alloys, acrylic, composite resin, ceramic, porcelain fused to metal, and gold (Fig. 11.7a, b).

Outcomes

The outcomes are dependent on the exactness of the procedures and the quality and quantity of underlying dentine [33]. These restorations require ongoing maintenance and monitoring and eventual replacement during adulthood. The primary goal in late childhood and adolescence should be to restore the teeth as effectively as possible to preserve tissue for subsequent restorations.

Conclusion

It can be very difficult for practitioners to decide how best to restore newly erupted permanent teeth that have hypomineralized or hypoplastic enamel. The primary aim is to protect the teeth from further breakdown and caries and to minimize sensitivity. In the anterior region, it is also important to address esthetic concerns. The second aim is to protect the pulp to allow normal maturation so that teeth will be permanently restorable in early adulthood. These goals are achievable using a combination of adhesive resin materials and preformed crowns including stainless steel crowns. These restorations can provide protection for up to 10 years during which time the developing occlusion can be managed in a multidisciplinary manner involving dentists, pediatric dentists, orthodontists, and prosthodontists. However, all this care is not without considerable cooperation from the child/young person. Practitioners should focus on providing the best interim solutions in the most acceptable way to the child and their family which may include accessing sedation and/or general anesthesia in addition to local anesthetic.

References

1. Dashash M, Yeung CA, Jamous I, Blinkhorn A. Interventions for the restorative care of amelogenesis imperfecta in children and adolescents. Cochrane Database Syst Rev. 2013;6:Cd007157.
2. Malik K, Gadhia K, Arkutu N, McDonald S, Blair F. The interdisciplinary management of patients with amelogenesis imperfecta – restorative dentistry. Br Dent J. 2012;212(11):537–42.
3. Munoz MA, Arana-Gordillo LA, Gomes GM, Gomes OM, Bombarda NH, Reis A, et al. Alternative esthetic management of fluorosis and hypoplasia stains: blending effect obtained with resin infiltration techniques. J Esthet Restor Dent. 2013;25(1):32–9.
4. Zagdwon AM, Fayle SA, Pollard MA. A prospective clinical trial comparing preformed metal crowns and cast restorations for defective first permanent molars. Eur J Paediatr Dent. 2003;4(3):138–42.
5. Lygidakis NA. Treatment modalities in children with teeth affected by molar-incisor enamel hypomineralisation (MIH): a systematic review. Eur Arch Paediatr Dent. 2010;11(2):65–74.
6. William V, Messer LB, Burrow MF. Molar incisor hypomineralization: review and recommendations for clinical management. Pediatr Dent. 2006;28(3):224–32.
7. Yamaguti PM, Acevedo AC, de Paula LM. Rehabilitation of an adolescent with autosomal dominant amelogenesis imperfecta: case report. Oper Dent. 2006;31(2):266–72.
8. William V, Burrow MF, Palamara JE, Messer LB. Microshear bond strength of resin composite to teeth affected by molar hypomineralization using 2 adhesive systems. Pediatr Dent. 2006;28(3):233–41.
9. Al-Sugair MH, Akpata ES. Effect of fluorosis on etching of human enamel. J Oral Rehabil. 1999;26(6):521–8.
10. Chay PL, Manton DJ, Palamara JE. The effect of resin infiltration and oxidative pre-treatment on microshear bond strength of resin composite to hypomineralised enamel. Int J Paediatr Dent. 2014;24(4):252–67.
11. Crombie F, Manton D, Palamara J, Reynolds E. Resin infiltration of developmentally hypomineralised enamel. Int J Paediatr Dent. 2014;24(1):51–5.
12. Gandhi S, Crawford P, Shellis P. The use of a 'bleach-etch-seal' deproteinization technique on MIH affected enamel. Int J Paediatr Dent. 2012;22(6):427–34.

13. Saroglu I, Aras S, Oztas D. Effect of deproteinization on composite bond strength in hypocalcified amelogenesis imperfecta. Oral Dis. 2006;12(3):305–8.
14. Torres-Gallegos I, Zavala-Alonso V, Patino-Marin N, Martinez-Castanon GA, Anusavice K, Loyola-Rodriguez JP. Enamel roughness and depth profile after phosphoric acid etching of healthy and fluorotic enamel. Aust Dent J. 2012;57(2):151–6.
15. Venezie RD, Vadiakas G, Christensen JR, Wright JT. Enamel pretreatment with sodium hypochlorite to enhance bonding in hypocalcified amelogenesis imperfecta: case report and SEM analysis. Pediatr Dent. 1994;16(6):433–6.
16. Marshman Z, Gibson B, Robinson PG. The impact of developmental defects of enamel on young people in the UK. Community Dent Oral Epidemiol. 2009;37(1):45–57.
17. Rodd HD, Abdul-Karim A, Yesudian G, O'Mahony J, Marshman Z. Seeking children's perspectives in the management of visible enamel defects. Int J Paediatr Dent. 2011;21(2):89–95.
18. Donly KJ, O'Neill M, Croll TP. Enamel microabrasion: a microscopic evaluation of the "abrosion effect". Quintessence Int. 1992;23(3):175–9.
19. Wray A, Welbury R. Treatment of intrinsic discolouration in permanent anterior teeth in children and adolescents. Available online at: www.rcseng.ac.uk. 2001; revised 2004. Accessed 2 Feb 2014.
20. Croll TP, Cavanaugh RR. Enamel color modification by controlled hydrochloric acid-pumice abrasion. I. Technique and examples. Quintessence Int. 1986;17(2):81–7.
21. Scherer W, Quattrone J, Chang J, David S, Vijayaraghavan T. Removal of intrinsic enamel stains with vital bleaching and modified microabrasion. Am J Dent. 1991;4(2):99–102.
22. Elkhazindar MM, Welbury RR. Enamel microabrasion. Dent Update. 2000;27(4):194–6.
23. Kilpatrick NM, Welbury RR. Hydrochloric acid/pumice microabrasion technique for the removal of enamel pigmentation. Dent Update. 1993;20(3):105–7.
24. Nathanson D. Vital tooth bleaching: sensitivity and pulpal considerations. J Am Dent Assoc. 1997;128(Suppl):41s–4.
25. Dadoun MP, Bartlett DW. Safety issues when using carbamide peroxide to bleach vital teeth–a review of the literature. Eur J Prosthodont Restor Dent. 2003;11(1):9–13.
26. Swift Jr EJ. Restorative considerations with vital tooth bleaching. J Am Dent Assoc. 1997;128(Suppl):60s–4.
27. Ritter AV, Leonard Jr RH, St Georges AJ, Caplan DJ, Haywood VB. Safety and stability of nightguard vital bleaching: 9 to 12 years post-treatment. J Esthet Restor Dent. 2002;14(5):275–85.
28. Welbury RR. A clinical study of a microfilled composite resin for labial veneers. Int J Paediatr Dent. 1991;1(1):9–15.
29. Ergun G, Kaya BM, Egilmez F, Cekic-Nagas I. Functional and esthetic rehabilitation of a patient with amelogenesis imperfecta. J Can Dent Assoc. 2013;79:d38.
30. Croll TP. Permanent molar stainless steel crown restoration. Quintessence Int. 1987;18(5):313–21.
31. Boj JR, Poirier C, Hernandez M, Espassa E, Espanya A. Case series: laser treatments for soft tissue problems in children. Eur Arch Paediatr Dent. 2011;12(2):113–7.
32. Rosenstiel S, Land M, Fujimoto J, editors. Contemporary fixed prosthodontics. 4th ed. St Louis: Mosby; 2006.
33. Harley KE, Ibbetson RJ. Dental anomalies–are adhesive castings the solution? Br Dent J. 1993;174(1):15–22.

Future Possibilities for Managing Dental Enamel Defects: Recent and Current Research Approaches

Agata Czajka-Jakubowska, Jun Liu, Sywe-Ren Chang, and Brian H. Clarkson

Abstract

The cause of an enamel defect can be genetic, systemic, local, and/or induced. The repair of these defects spans the fields from gene therapy to invasive or non-invasive conventional restorative therapies. No matter how disfiguring some of the genetic and systemic conditions are, it is unlikely that the modern techniques of genetic and tissue engineering will be used in the near future to repair or prevent these enamel defects. Clinicians will have to rely on more conventional invasive, minimally invasive, and noninvasive techniques to treat this problem. This chapter describes some new and novel techniques which are in use and/or development for the repair of enamel defects. They include: growing enamel crystals on dental substrates, penetration of carious lesions with self-assembling molecules which encourage mineral formation, infiltrating carious lesions with resins, a paint on "enamel" using a self-etch resin, and an "enamel" crystal containing flexible laminate – a tooth "Band-Aid."

Disclaimer The technology for the products described in the latter part of the chapter has been licensed from the University of Michigan to a spin-off company, TruEnmel, of which the authors are part owners.

A. Czajka-Jakubowska, PhD
Department of Maxillofacial Orthopedics and Orthodontics,
Poznan University of Medical Sciences, Poznan, Poland
e-mail: czajak@it.pl

J. Liu, PhD • S.-R. Chang, MS • B.H. Clarkson, BChD, MS, PhD (✉)
Department of Cariology, Restorative Sciences and Endodontics,
School of Dentistry, University of Michigan, Ann Arbor, MI 48103, USA
e-mail: junlc@umich.edu; renchang@umich.edu;
bricla@umich.edu

© Springer-Verlag Berlin Heidelberg 2015
B.K. Drummond, N. Kilpatrick (eds.), *Planning and Care for Children
and Adolescents with Dental Enamel Defects: Etiology, Research
and Contemporary Management*, DOI 10.1007/978-3-662-44800-7_12

Introduction

There are a wide range of putative causes of development defects of enamel (DDE) including: genetic, for example, amelogenesis imperfecta (AI); systemic, which causes a generalized disturbance of enamel formation, as in fluorosis; or local disturbances causing hypoplasia. The etiology of DDE has been discussed in great detail in Chaps. 1, 2, 3, 4, and 5. There are also acquired enamel defects, or those which can be loosely defined as defects resulting from a disease, such as caries or caused iatrogenically during the repair of a disease. Other acquired defects may include cracks, abfractions, wear, and erosion. The potential to repair these defects ranges from very complex gene therapy to the more conventional, invasive restorative techniques. In the near future, it is expected that several forms of noninvasive restorative therapy will become routine.

Genetic Engineering

Using genetic engineering to "cure" a genetic disturbance of enamel no matter how disfiguring is unlikely in the short term until this technology is perfected on lethal diseases and declared safe. Reports of bioengineered tooth development, including successfully using differentiated stem cells to produce dental enamel and "teeth," suggest that in time, this technology may be mastered for clinical use [1]. However, the issue of whether such "engineered" teeth can achieve useful function is another area of research that will require significant effort. Function would include normal enamel appearance especially in the anterior region, masticatory function, compatibility with other tissues, and neurological responsiveness via the dentin to allow the teeth to respond to stimuli in the oral cavity. One line of research has been focusing on identifying specific cellular pathways that are affected by genetic mutations resulting in altered amelogenesis (or enamel formation) leading to the eruption of teeth with hypomineralized or hypoplastic enamel. Many such mutations have now been identified, and our understanding of how each mutation affects the cellular pathways is evolving. In at least one case, a mutation in the gene encoding the principle developing enamel matrix protein, amelogenin, appears to result in protein misfolding or premature aggregation such that it cannot be processed through the normal cellular secretory pathways resulting in what is described as a "cell stress" response. This can eventually cause apoptosis (cell death) [2]. Recent research of a particular mutation in mice that results in defective enamel similar to that occurring in human AI suggests that there may be opportunities to "rescue" the pathway in several different ways. Brookes and co-workers [3] have shown rescue of the enamel phenotype in female mice with an amelogenin mutation by a drug (sodium phenylbutyrate) that supports the cells to avoid apoptosis and thus go on to complete enamel formation. This is a promising approach that has already been shown to improve outcomes in other human diseases caused by particular mutations that invoke cell stress. This line of enquiry in enamel development still requires many years of research to translate into clinical use in humans. However, it has the potential to successfully improve enamel formation in permanent teeth if the problem can be identified at birth or in the first few months of life. This would be possible given a known family history. However, for many children AI is not diagnosed until the permanent teeth start to erupt, and so this particular approach might only benefit some of the later developing teeth.

One of the problems of using another recent medical technology, tissue engineering to develop new enamel, is that this is only applicable to tissues with living cells. Unfortunately, the ameloblast undergoes apoptosis and dies once enamel has reached maturity. This makes enamel regeneration impossible unless a source of a person's stem cells could be engineered or redirected to produce viable ameloblasts. While this has been shown to be possible in in vitro conditions, how this enamel could be used to "restore" enamel in erupted teeth remains a challenge. Therefore, it is believed that the more conventional ways of treating defective enamel will continue for the foreseeable future.

Enamel Crystal Development

Growing biomimetic enamel crystals, both in vitro and in vivo, has been shown to be possible by a number of scientific groups [4–10]. Studies have reported using enamel proteins (amelogenin) [5, 6, 8], peptides and artificial proteins [11], and dendrimers [4, 10] to promote the growth of fluorhydroxyapatite (FHA) on etched enamel surfaces. Other studies have used pure chemical solutions in an attempt to grow enamel-like structures on etched enamel surfaces. Perhaps the most convincing of these is that reported by Yin et al. in 2009 [12]. They were able, after 8 days and near physiological conditions, to grow enamel-like crystals on etched human enamel surfaces. The FHA crystal had the characteristic shape of human enamel crystals and a calcium/phosphorus ratio of 1.59 similar to the expected ratio of FHA of 1.67. However, whether the crystal growth would have occurred in the presence of saliva which contains crystal growth inhibitors including statherin is debatable. The artificial protein, polyamidoamine dendrimers (PAMAM) have been used as scaffolds for enamel-like crystal growth in both in vitro and in vivo studies [4, 10]. The PAMAM dendrimers are modified with carboxylic acid groups (COOH) that allows them to be adsorbed onto etched enamel surfaces where they act as a template for enamel-like crystal formation. Further modification with alendronate (ALN) increases the binding strength to the etched enamel. These modified dendrimers were used in an in vivo study where they were adsorbed onto enamel sections and sewn to the inside of rat cheeks [10]. After 28 days, the sections were removed, and enamel coatings analyzed. The coatings had a calcium/phosphorous ratio of 1.67 identical to the ratio of human enamel apatite, but the images of the crystals did not show the normal morphology of human enamel crystals. Enamel-like crystals have been successfully grown on various substrates, dentin, the amelodentinal junction, and metal (implant) surfaces [13]. Thus, this technology is available, but problems do exist when attempting to translate it for *in vivo* use. The crystals grow slowly; there is low strength of adhesion of the crystals to the substrate; and the crystals have to be protected during their growth phase from the forces of mastication, tooth brushing, hot and cold drinks, and occasionally the low pH of these drinks.

Another approach has been to infiltrate demineralized lesions with self-assembling peptides [11]. These peptides then self-assemble to produce a molecule that attracts calcium, resulting in laying down mineral within the subsurface lesion. Recently, a clinical trial demonstrated the remineralization potential of these peptides [14]. Translating this approach to improving hypomineralized enamel presents different problems that are related to the increased and different types of protein in the lesions, but future research is expected to overcome the problems of the protein and allow improvement of mineral-deficient enamel.

A somewhat different approach that combines repair and caries prevention has been investigated. It focuses on the concept of noninvasive dentistry. The concept is based on the knowledge that caries is caused by bacteria which die or at least become quiescent once deprived of nourishment. Thus, there is no need to remove diseased demineralized or hypomineralized enamel or carious dentin, as long as the bacteria are deprived of any nutrients. This effect of sealing bacteria in tissue has been reported in several studies over the past 30 years or more, the classic being the study of Mertz-Fairhurst et al. [15]. This study clearly showed that carious dentin left in teeth which had been completely sealed, thus depriving the bacteria of nourishment, did not show caries progression after 10 years. The success of sealing teeth, the difficulty in deciding when to re-restore, and an understanding of the damage to teeth caused by re-restoration of teeth should be strong influences in supporting the concept of noninvasive restorative dentistry [16]. It should awaken dentistry from its scientific slumber and base the management of diseased dental tissues on current and new scientific and clinical evidence and not just remain reliant on the teaching and practices of the past.

Two recent technologies "filling without drilling," which purport to be noninvasive, do in fact have a degree of invasiveness because they require the removal of the surface layer of non-cavitated demineralized enamel lesions by acid etching to allow penetration of the lesion by the material being used. One of these, DMG Icon low viscosity resin, is already in clinical use, and the outcomes of a clinical trial of the other, using self-assembling peptides, have recently been reported. The Icon technology marketed by DMG involves etching the enamel surface with hydrochloric acid which allows infiltration of the subsurface lesion with a low viscosity resin which is then cured thus sealing the defect [17, 18]. However, this technique of infiltration has not yet been demonstrated to be as successful in hypomineralized lesions [19]. The other technology using self-assembling peptide molecules to infiltrate the lesion and promote remineralization has been described above [11, 14, 20]. Both of these technologies are an improvement on the "drill and fill" approach which is still very common in dentistry today, and it is hoped that similar technologies will be able to be utilized for hypomineralized lesions in the future.

Researchers have considered that the approach using low viscosity resin like the Icon technique could be improved by the introduction of enamel-like nanocrystals into the resin prior to the application of the resin, therefore producing an enamel-like crystal-filled subsurface lesion. Another biochemical application, in contrast to the self-assembling peptides, is to use a phosphoprotein or a phosphorylated peptide like serine. This protein or peptide having infiltrated the carious lesion, either in

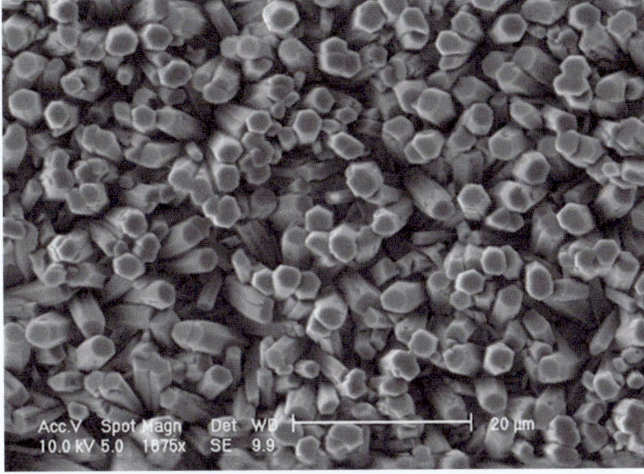

Fig. 12.1 FHA crystals synthesized under hydrothermal conditions

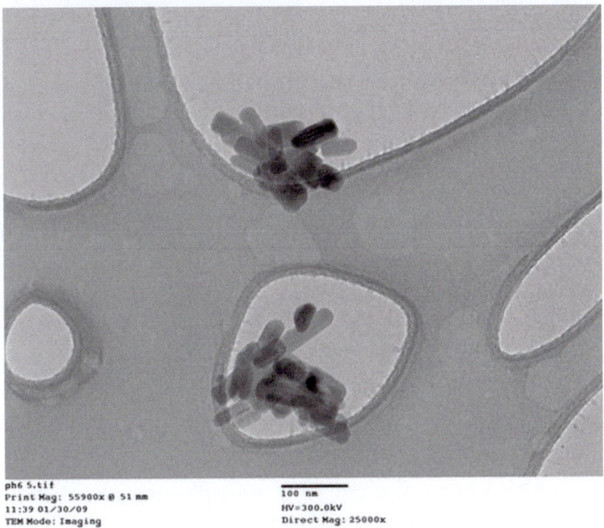

Fig. 12.2 FHA crystals synthesized under ambient conditions

enamel or dentin, would "catalyze" the formation of mineral from plaque fluid and/or saliva [21].

In 2006, a landmark paper by Chen et al. described the in vitro synthesis of FHA crystals and their ability to coat a substrate with these crystals which had a prism-like structure resembling the surface of human enamel [22]. The effects of these coatings on the *in vitro* and *in vivo* response of various cell lines have been reported [23–25]. In 2013, Clark et al. reported the anticariogenic effect of FHA coated preformed stainless steel crowns at the tooth/crown margin in an in vitro model [26]. These enamel-like crystals and coatings are synthesized without the use of cells or proteins. They can be produced under hydrothermal (Fig. 12.1) or ambient conditions (Fig. 12.2). The crystals resemble enamel crystals in shape, composition, and size. The larger FHA crystals seen in Fig. 12.1 are produced by applying heat and a

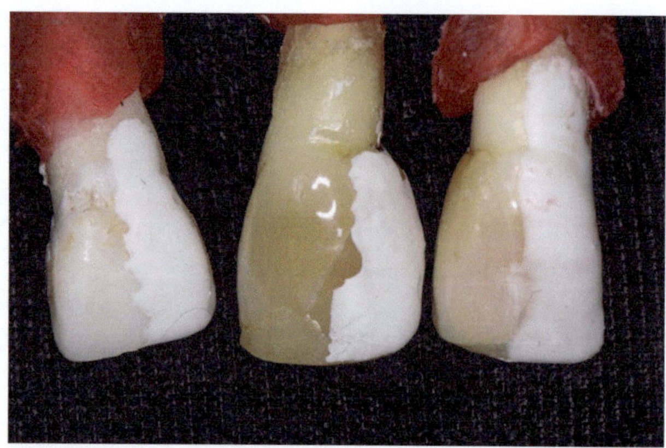

Fig. 12.3 "Paint on enamel" for the treatment of enamel defects including early carious lesions. It can also be tinted to match the tooth color or in this case to whiten discolored teeth. Right half of the tooth was painted with self-etch adhesive plus FHA crystals and titanium dioxide

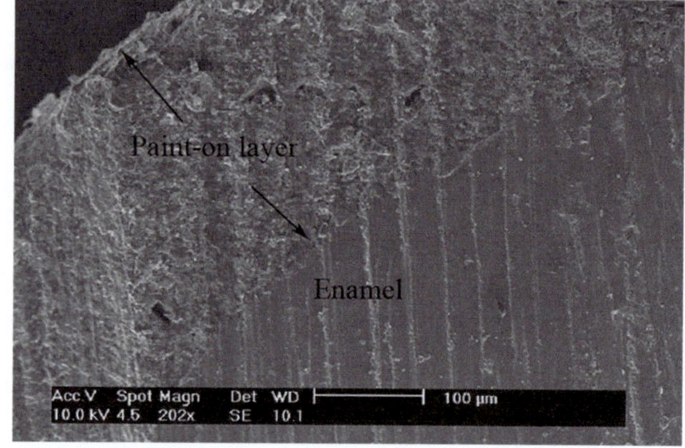

Fig. 12.4 SEM observation of the "paint on enamel" layer on the enamel surface showing the intimacy of contact between the "paint on enamel" and the tooth

small amount of pressure for 10 h. The crystals synthesized under ambient conditions are smaller and take up to 1–3 days to form. All the crystals are produced from a solution containing calcium, phosphorus, and fluoride. Irrespective of how they are synthesized, the crystals have a calcium/phosphorus ratio of approximately 1.67, the same as human enamel crystals, and an x-ray diffraction pattern typical of FHA [27].

The crystals have been incorporated into several different vehicles including resins, a laboratory-synthesized substance that resembles the "glue" that allows mollusks to adhere to rocks in the ocean and water. Variations of these mixtures could be used in the treatment and prevention of caries, tooth sensitivity, and erosion or to "whiten" discolored teeth. An ideal vehicle for the FHA crystals might be any of the self-etch adhesives which are now used routinely in dentistry. The concept is that this combination can be used as a "paint on" enamel. Because of the acid nature of the adhesive, it will bond to enamel and dentin allowing it to cover those surfaces with a layer of enamel crystals. It can be tinted to match the color of the tooth or to whiten a discolored tooth (Fig. 12.3). It could also be used to repair carious and erosive lesions (Fig. 12.4), as an occlusal sealant (Fig. 12.5) or as desensitizing

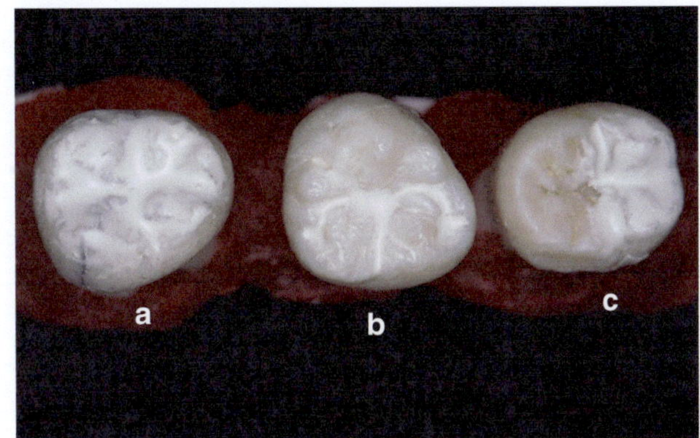

Fig. 12.5 "Paint on enamel" to seal molar occlusal surfaces. (**a**) Whole occlusal surface sealed. (**b**) Fissures only sealed. (**c**) Right half occlusal surface sealed

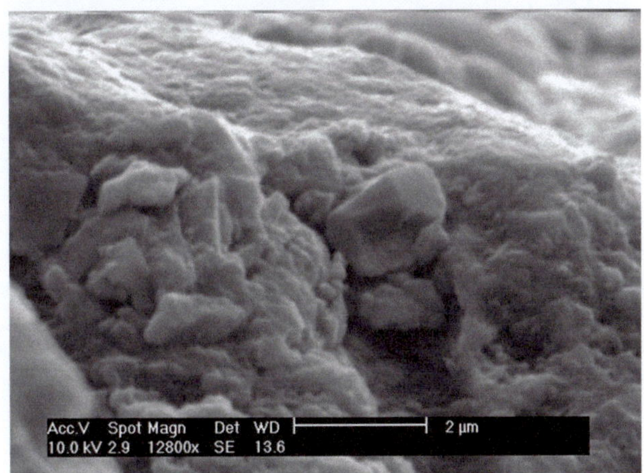

Fig. 12.6 SEM image of "paint on enamel" occluding a dentinal tubule

Fig. 12.7 Fluoride release from a bis-GMA/TEGDMA composite of different filler % vol. of unsilanated and silanated FHA crystals for 1 day, 1 week, and 1 month

Composite	1 day F, ppm	1wk F, ppm	1 mo F, ppm
bisGMA/TEGDMA with 75% silanated silica	0.07	0.08	0.06
bisGMA/TEGDMA w/ 63% unsilanated FA	0.8	2.1	1.3
bisGMA/TEGDMA w/ 42% silanated silica & 20% silanated FA	0.1	0.3	0.5

agent (Fig. 12.6) – a five-in-one product. One further advantage of this technology is that it will release fluoride over time even if incorporated into a resin (Fig. 12.7). This will allow not only the treatment options described above but may also have a caries-preventive effect by promoting remineralization or possibly continuing

Fig. 12.8 Flexural strength and elastic modulus (%) of a bis-GMA/TEGDMA composite filled with silanated silica (Ssilica) particles and nonsilanated FA (NSFHA) crystals

Composite fill (%)	Flexural Strength (Mpa)	Elastic Modulus (Gpa)
100 Ssilica	126±26	6.2±1.9
10 (NSFOHA) 90 Ssilica	90±23	8.9±4.0
20 (NSFOHA) 80 Ssilica	118±22	7.8±2.7

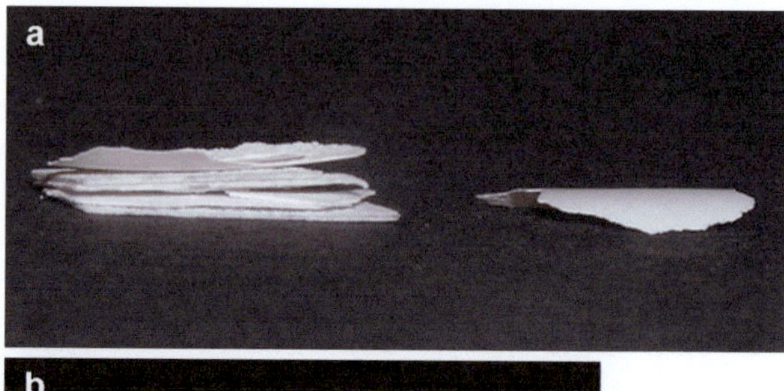
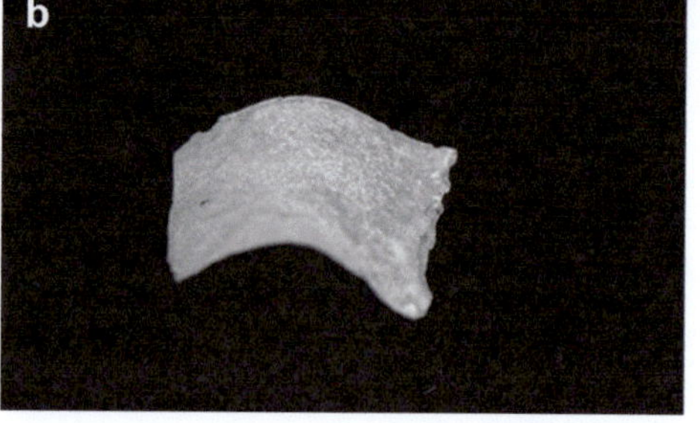

Fig. 12.9 (**a**) Brittle FHA films and (**b**) pliable FHA/Euradgit films

mineralization in teeth which are hypomineralized at eruption such as those with hypomineralized AI or MIH a though this has yet to be established. Large structural defects could be restored with a composite material that is partially filled with the FHA crystals (Fig. 12.8). As can be seen in Fig. 12.8, the mechanical properties of the composite material are not diminished if FHA crystals are substituted for 20 % of the silanated silica. This "paint on" enamel technology again promotes the concept of noninvasive dentistry where it can be applied over early demineralized lesions on smooth or occlusal surfaces. Further research is now required to evaluate this technology in in vivo settings and clinical trials.

It has also been shown that the FHA crystals can be produced as a film (Fig. 12.9), but these tend to be brittle and unsuitable for use as laminates. It is thought that laminates could have a temporary role in protecting lesions, including hypomineralized lesions, while they are mineralizing. In order to obtain a flexible

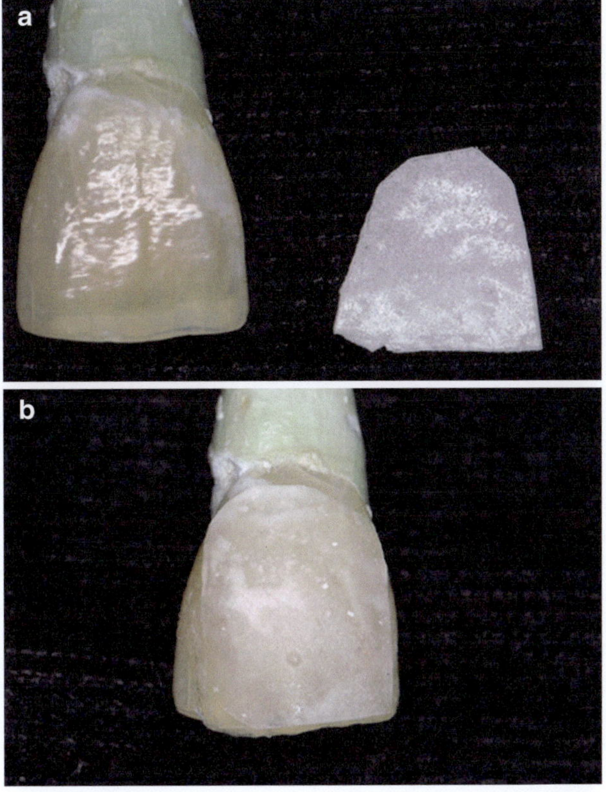

Fig. 12.10 (**a**) Human incisor tooth and FHA/Euradgit laminate and (**b**) FHA/Euradgit laminate applied to the buccal surface of human incisor tooth

laminate which would conform to the curved surface of a tooth, the crystals have been mixed with a polymer with the trade name of Eudragit. This is used as an enteric coating for tablets (e.g., aspirin) and it dissolves at various pHs. It has the advantage of being approved by the Federal Drug Administration in the USA for use in humans. This laminate is white in appearance and is flexible (Fig. 12.10a). It can be cut to any size and is easily adapted to the curved surface of a tooth. It can be bonded to the tooth surface, or, if allowed to dry on the tooth, it will adhere to that surface. It could be used like a "Band-Aid" to cover discolored, defective enamel and early carious lesions without removing any tooth tissue. The laminate is esthetic and will cover large areas of tooth surface (Fig. 12.10b). It is hoped that as the Eudragit dissolves over time, the FHA crystals will become incorporated into the enamel surface producing a surface with high-fluoride content. This laminate will achieve an esthetic repair along with caries-preventive activity – a noninvasive approach.

The latter part of this chapter has described two potential products for the repair and prevention of enamel defects. Prototypes of these modalities have already been tested *in vitro* and are good examples of potential noninvasive type of products. There is now the need for them to undergo clinical testing to establish their usefulness in clinical practice.

Conclusion

It can be seen from current research approaches that the future will hold many new approaches to managing teeth not only with enamel defects but also with defects created by dental caries and dental trauma of various kinds. The approaches will be influenced by improved understanding of genetic effects at the cellular level and by how these might be modified. They will also be influenced by the development of biomimetic materials for use throughout the body. This will require dental practitioners to engage with the new technologies and to embrace the evolving understanding of dental hard tissues in health and disease. To do this, the profession needs to continue to move from a primarily restorative approach to treating diseases of the dental hard tissues that involves removal of damaged tissue to one which alters and modifies the tissues even when defective.

References

1. Ikeda E, Morita R, Nakao K, Ishida K, Nakamura T, Takano-Yamamoto T, et al. Fully functional bioengineered tooth replacement as an organ replacement therapy. Proc Natl Acad Sci U S A. 2009;106(32):13475–80.
2. Barron MJ, Brookes SJ, Kirkham J, Shore RC, Hunt C, Mironov A, et al. A mutation in the mouse Amelx tri-tyrosyl domain results in impaired secretion of amelogenin and phenocopies human X-linked amelogenesis imperfecta. Hum Mol Genet. 2010;19(7):1230–47.
3. Brookes SJ, Barron MJ, Boot-Handford R, Kirkham J, Dixon MJ. Endoplasmic reticulum stress in amelogenesis imperfecta and phenotypic rescue using 4-phenylbutyrate. Hum Mol Genet. 2014;23(9):2468–80.
4. Chen L, Liang K, Li J, Wu D, Zhou X, Li J. Regeneration of biomimetic hydroxyapatite on etched human enamel by anionic PAMAM template in vitro. Arch Oral Biol. 2013;58(8):975–80.
5. Habelitz S, DenBesten PK, Marshall SJ, Marshall GW, Li W. Self-assembly and effect on crystal growth of the leucine-rich amelogenin peptide. Eur J Oral Sci. 2006;114 Suppl 1:315–9. Discussion 27 – 9, 82.
6. Habelitz S, Kullar A, Marshall SJ, DenBesten PK, Balooch M, Marshall GW, et al. Amelogenin-guided crystal growth on fluoroapatite glass-ceramics. J Dent Res. 2004;83(9):698–702.
7. Ishikawa K, Eanes ED, Tung MS. The effect of supersaturation on apatite crystal formation in aqueous solutions at physiologic pH and temperature. J Dent Res. 1994;73(8):1462–9.
8. Uskokovic V, Li W, Habelitz S. Biomimetic precipitation of uniaxially grown calcium phosphate crystals from full-length human amelogenin sols. J Bionic Eng. 2011;8(2):114–21.
9. Wang X, Xia C, Zhang Z, Deng X, Wei S, Zheng G, et al. Direct growth of human enamel-like calcium phosphate microstructures on human tooth. J Nanosci Nanotechnol. 2009;9(2):1361–4.

10. Wu D, Yang J, Li J, Chen L, Tang B, Chen X, et al. Hydroxyapatite-anchored dendrimer for in situ remineralization of human tooth enamel. Biomaterials. 2013;34(21):5036–47.
11. Kirkham J, Firth A, Vernals D, Boden N, Robinson C, Shore RC, et al. Self-assembling peptide scaffolds promote enamel remineralization. J Dent Res. 2007;86(5):426–30.
12. Yin Y, Yun S, Fang J, Chen H. Chemical regeneration of human tooth enamel under near-physiological conditions. Chem Commun (Camb). 2009 (39):5892–4.
13. Czajka-Jakubowska AE, Liu J, Chang SR, Clarkson BH. The effect of the surface characteristics of various substrates on fluorapatite crystal growth, alignment, and spatial orientation. Med Sci Monit. 2009;15(6):Mt84–8.
14. Brunton PA, Davies RP, Burke JL, Smith A, Aggeli A, Brookes SJ, et al. Treatment of early caries lesions using biomimetic self-assembling peptides–a clinical safety trial. Br Dent J. 2013;215(4):E6.
15. Mertz-Fairhurst EJ, Curtis Jr JW, Ergle JW, Rueggeberg FA, Adair SM. Ultraconservative and cariostatic sealed restorations: results at year 10. J Am Dent Assoc. 1998;129(1):55–66.
16. Anusavice KJ. Treatment regimens in preventive and restorative dentistry. J Am Dent Assoc. 1995;126(6):727–43.
17. Meyer-Lueckel H, Paris S. Improved resin infiltration of natural caries lesions. J Dent Res. 2008;87(12):1112–6.
18. Rocha Gomes Torres C, Borges AB, Torres LM, Gomes IS, de Oliveira RS. Effect of caries infiltration technique and fluoride therapy on the colour masking of white spot lesions. J Dent. 2011;39(3):202–7.
19. Crombie F, Manton D, Palamara J, Reynolds E. Resin infiltration of developmentally hypo-mineralised enamel. Int J Paediatr Dent. 2014;24(1):51–5.
20. Firth A, Aggeli A, Burke JL, Yang X, Kirkham J. Biomimetic self-assembling peptides as injectable scaffolds for hard tissue engineering. Nanomedicine (Lond). 2006;1(2):189–99.
21. Chang S, Chen H, Liu J, Wood D, Bentley P, Clarkson B. Synthesis of a potentially bioactive, hydroxyapatite-nucleating molecule. Calcif Tissue Int. 2006;78(1):55–61.
22. Chen H, Tang Z, Liu J, Sun K, Chang SR, Peters MC, et al. Acellular synthesis of a human enamel-like microstructure. Adv Mater. 2006;18(14):1846–51.
23. Liu J, Jin T, Chang S, Czajka-Jakubowska A, Zhang Z, Nor JE, et al. The effect of novel fluorapatite surfaces on osteoblast-like cell adhesion, growth, and mineralization. Tissue Eng Part A. 2010;16(9):2977–86.
24. Liu J, Jin TC, Chang S, Czajka-Jakubowska A, Clarkson BH. Adhesion and growth of dental pulp stem cells on enamel-like fluorapatite surfaces. J Biomed Mater Res A. 2011;96(3):528–34.
25. Liu J, Wang X, Jin Q, Jin T, Chang S, Zhang Z, et al. The stimulation of adipose-derived stem cell differentiation and mineralization by ordered rod-like fluorapatite coatings. Biomaterials. 2012;33(20):5036–46.
26. Clark DR, Czajka-Jakubowska A, Rick C, Liu J, Chang S, Clarkson BH. In vitro anti-caries effect of fluoridated hydroxyapatite-coated preformed metal crowns. Eur Arch Paediatr Dent. 2013;14(4):253–8.
27. Chen H, Sun K, Tang Z, Law RV, Mansfield JF, Clarkson BH. Synthesis of fluorapatite nanorods and nanowires by direct precipitation from solution. Cryst Growth Des. 2006;6(6):1504–8.

Final Comments

13

Bernadette K. Drummond and Nicky Kilpatrick

Abstract

This chapter sums up the information provided by an international group of authors on dental enamel defects (DDE) in children and adolescents. It comments on the difficulty of identifying defects in individuals based on indices that have been developed for prevalence studies. It comments on the significant impact DDE have on quality of life and notes the difficulties in providing care that exists because of limited evidence of outcomes from different procedures. Finally it encourages clinicians to work with dental specialists in early childhood to plan the best available path to the permanent dentition.

Developmental defects of enamel (DDE) account for an apparent increasingly large burden of dental treatment required in children and adolescents. Despite a plethora of studies and overwhelming anecdotal clinical reports, there remain difficulties and wide variation in describing and defining these defects. There are limitations in all of the reported indices which, while useful in epidemiological studies, are often not appropriate in the clinical setting when trying to understand or diagnose DDE in an individual case. Currently, even when a label is assigned to a particular type of defect, it often does not indicate the treatment approach that should be followed. This is best illustrated by Molar Incisor Hypomineralization (MIH) which, has been recognized for many years but only recently identified as a unique DDE condition and as such, still has no defined management path. There have been many reports

B.K. Drummond, BDS, MS, PhD (✉)
Department of Oral Sciences, Faculty of Dentistry, University of Otago,
310 Great King Street, PO Box 647, Dunedin 9054, New Zealand
e-mail: bernadette.drummond@otago.ac.nz

N. Kilpatrick, BDS, PhD
Cleft and Craniofacial Research, Murdoch Childrens Research Institute,
Flemington Road, Parkville, Melbourne, VIC 3052, Australia
e-mail: nicky@bassdata.com.au

© Springer-Verlag Berlin Heidelberg 2015
B.K. Drummond, N. Kilpatrick (eds.), *Planning and Care for Children and Adolescents with Dental Enamel Defects: Etiology, Research and Contemporary Management*, DOI 10.1007/978-3-662-44800-7_13

describing the structure and composition of the compromised enamel in the different presentations of DDE. More recently, reports describing the genetic influences, including specific mutations, linked to different types of DDE have been appearing in the literature. However, management remains a very real challenge for clinicians and patients alike. While there are many case reports of clinical management of DDE, there is still no good evidence for proven successful ways to manage DDE in very young children or through adolescence until permanent restorative solutions can be provided.

With these considerations in mind, this book has been written by a group of authors, colleagues, and friends, all of whom have wide experience investigating and managing DDE. The aims are to summarize what is currently known about the prevalence and etiology of DDE and to provide guidance for clinicians when faced with managing DDE in children and adolescents. We hope to encourage interest in providing care for these children and adolescents to allow them to reach adulthood as confident young people with healthy smiles and functioning dentitions. The growing awareness of the broader impacts of DDE on young people, and in particular their oral health-related quality of life, has been recognized and is reviewed. Where the defects involve anterior teeth, appearance is compromised which has a significant impact on the affected individual particularly when other children or adults comment on their "different" teeth. Furthermore, defective enamel is often sensitive with young children complaining they cannot eat ice cream. It follows that oral hygiene and tooth brushing in particular is likely compromised and prevention of dental caries may be more difficult. Options for decreasing sensitivity to help with preventive care are discussed.

Unlike caries, there is still no good evidence to support reliable approaches to the management of different types of DDE during childhood. This book presents a range of options for maintaining the primary and young permanent dentitions throughout childhood. These options include optimizing appearance, in terms of both the color and shape of teeth as well as the occlusion; reducing sensitivity; maintaining function; minimizing wear and caries as well as promoting healthy periodontal tissues; and most importantly of all helping these young people to develop dental coping skills for the long-term complex restorative care that may be required well in to adulthood.

This book has drawn on the experience, skills, and research outcomes from dental clinicians and researchers across the world. It has allowed these writers to summarize their knowledge and to challenge others to think about and realize their role in recognizing DDE, recording what they see, and ensuring, where appropriate, that these dental problems are recorded alongside any other general health problems. In this way dental professionals can contribute to advancing understanding of the links between genetic/medical conditions and DDE which will, in turn, inform development of technological approaches to rescuing teeth before the defects develop.

We hope that readers will be able to use the information in this book in their management of DDE and that they will continue to seek better restorative solutions for these problems and collaborate with specialists including pediatric dentists, orthodontists, prosthodontists and researchers in tooth development to allow patients and parents to have a long-term vision of healthy and functional smiles in adulthood.

Index

© Springer-Verlag Berlin Heidelberg 2015
B.K. Drummond, N. Kilpatrick (eds.), *Planning and Care for Children
and Adolescents with Dental Enamel Defects: Etiology, Research
and Contemporary Management,* DOI 10.1007/978-3-662-44800-7